チーム医療のための メディカル英語 基本表現100

[編著] 髙木久代・小澤淑子

講談社

はじめに

　現代社会では医療がますます複雑になり，それに伴い医療の高度化と専門性の分化が進んでいます．そのため，医療は各分野の専門家たちとともに行う「チーム医療」へ変わってきました．
「チーム医療」に携わる医師，看護師，薬剤師，放射線技師，理学療法士，臨床検査技師，管理栄養士，鍼灸師などは今まで以上に相互理解を深め，さらに尊重することが求められています．本書は英語で「病院内の各診療科における病気と治療」を学ぶことによって，医療人が共有すべき専門知識を習得していただき，さらに在学中のみならず卒業後も医学英語論文により高度な医療知識を習得するために英語力が必要な学生たちが，将来医療現場で使える基本的な英語語彙，英語表現を学ぶことを目的としています．
　また医療と英語に興味のある方にも，本書を通して英語で基礎的な医学知識を習得していただき，海外での病気治療時や，日本を訪問する外国人の病気対応時などに役立てていただきたいと思います．
　本書を活用し，医療分野での互いの理解と尊敬を深め，英語力のさらなる向上がなされることを願っております．
　最後に，本書を出版することができましたのは講談社サイエンティフィクの三浦洋一郎様をはじめ，皆様のご支援によるところが大きく，心より感謝申し上げます．また，米国人の立場から様々なご助言をしていただいた鈴鹿医療科学大学の Mark LaForge 氏にも感謝申し上げます．

2015 年 2 月
著者一同

本書の特長

1. 本書は，加藤家，三浦家を中心とした人々を登場させ，病院内での，①各診療科における病気と治療，②病気と治療にかかわる医療専門家に関する話題を全15章で取り上げています。また，2章から13章までは，病気とその治療にかかわる医療専門家を，「2章と3章」「4章と5章」というように2章ごとに連携する章で取り上げていますので，**興味のある2章ごと**に利用していただくことができます。
2. 各章のMedical Dialogue（医療会話）の中で，医療現場で重要な「100の医療表現（Medical Expressions）」を記載してあります。記載されている**表現を何度も読み，完全に覚えましょう**。
3. 言葉をもつ人間社会において，互いのコミュニケーションは重要です。特に医療現場では，医師と患者，患者と看護師などの関係をスムーズに保ち，より良い治療を実践するにはコミュニケーションの能力が求められます。各章の「Let's Use Communication Strategies!」で会話の具体例を学ぶことで，**コミュニケーション能力の改善**を導くことができます。
4. 各章の「Medical Dialogue（医療会話）」「Medical Reading（医療英文）」「Medical Terminology（医療専門用語）」を学ぶことにより，論文読解，医療カルテの理解に役立てることができます。
5. 各章にある「Helpful English Grammar（役に立つ英文法）」は医療分野の論文や記事の理解に必要な英文法です。よく理解するようにしましょう。

各章の構成

1. **Medical Dialogue** ▶基本医療表現，医療専門用語，会話文が含まれています。会話文は，病院での医師と患者，看護師と患者など，医療専門家と患者との診察，治療などの会話で成り立っています。
2. **Let's Use Communication Strategies!** ▶コミュニケーション能力を向上させましょう。
3. **Medical Reading** ▶疾病，治療，医療専門家の仕事などについて学びます。
4. **Comprehension** ▶ Medical Readingについての理解を問う問題です。
5. **Helpful English Grammar** ▶基本となる英文法を理解しましょう。
6. **ほっと一息！** ▶医療分野に関わるちょっとためになる話題を提供しています。

Medical DialogueとMedical Readingの和訳は，弊社ホームページ（http://www.kspub.co.jp/book/）に掲載しています。

目次

はじめに　　　　　　　　　　　　　　　　　　　　　　　　　iii

Chapter 1
Japanese National Health Insurance and Medical Sheet
日本の医療保険と問診表　　　　　　　　　　　　　　　　　　1

Chapter 2
Internal Medicine: Influenza
内科：インフルエンザ　　　　　　　　　　　　　　　　　　　12

Chapter 3
Nurse
看護師　　　　　　　　　　　　　　　　　　　　　　　　　　23

Chapter 4
Internal Medicine: Hepatic Disease
内科：肝炎　　　　　　　　　　　　　　　　　　　　　　　　33

Chapter 5
Blood Test: Medical Technologist
血液検査：臨床検査技師　　　　　　　　　　　　　　　　　　44

Chapter 6
Internal Medicine: Diabetes
内科：糖尿病　　　　　　　　　　　　　　　　　　　　　　　56

Chapter 7
Diabetes and Registered Dietitian
糖尿病と管理栄養士　　　　　　　　　　　　　　　　　　　　69

Chapter 8
Orthopedics: Traumatic Fracture
整形外科：外傷性骨折　　　　　　　　　　　　　　　　　　　81

Chapter 9
Rehabilitation: Physical Therapist
リハビリテーション：理学療法士　　　　　　　　　　　　　92

Chapter 10
Further Examination of the Lung:
Lung Cancer
肺の精密検査：肺がん　　　　　　　　　　　　　　　　　104

Chapter 11
PET-CT Scan:
Medical Radiation Technologist
PET-CTスキャン：診療放射線技師　　　　　　　　　　　　116

Chapter 12
Pediatrics: Bronchial Asthma
小児科：気管支喘息　　　　　　　　　　　　　　　　　　128

Chapter 13
Medication for a Young Child:
Pharmacist
小児の薬物療法：薬剤師　　　　　　　　　　　　　　　　140

Chapter 14
Acupuncture and Acupuncturist
鍼灸と鍼灸師　　　　　　　　　　　　　　　　　　　　　152

Chapter 15
Hemodialysis:
Interdisciplinary Team Approach to Medicine
血液透析：チーム医療　　　　　　　　　　　　　　　　　164

Comprehension　解答　　　　　　　　　　　　　　　　176

索引　　　　　　　　　　　　　　　　　　　　　　　　180

イラスト：MINOMURA

本書に登場する人たち

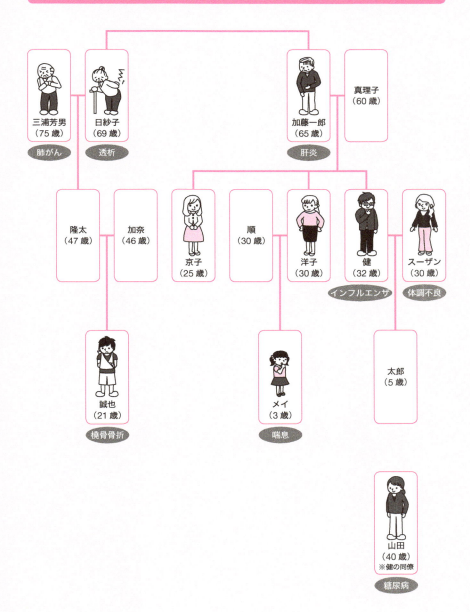

Chapter 1
Japanese National Health Insurance and Medical Sheet

日本の医療保険と問診表

日本の医療制度と他の国の医療制度は異なっています。会話から医療制度の違いを学びましょう。問診表に書かれている医療専門語彙を学び，問診表に記入しましょう。

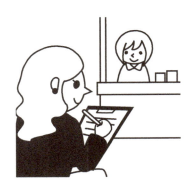

Purposes of this Chapter

臨床英語表現	日本の医療保険に関する表現
コミュニケーション・ストラテジー	発言全体を聞き直す
医療従事者の知識	問診表内の英語語彙学習，問診表記入
重要構文	They say ～，現在完了，the former ～ the latter ～，指示代名詞の that

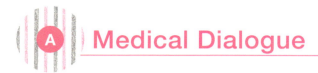
Medical Dialogue

Basic Medical Expressions

医療現場でよく使われる簡単な表現です。自然に言えるようになるまで声に出して何度も読み，完全に覚えましょう。

---

1 Has your fever gone down already?
熱はもう下がりましたか？

現在完了の英文で，完了を示しています。

---

2 I feel sluggish with a slight fever.
熱が少しあり，体がだるい。

高熱は a high fever です。fever は発熱状態で，temperature は体温を示します。

---

3 I have had a slight fever for some time.
近頃微熱があります。

have ＋過去分詞の現在完了の英文で，「ずっと～している」と継続を示しています。
動作が継続する場合，現在完了進行形の方がより継続を表現することができます。
（**I have been cleaning** my room for three hours. 3 時間**ずっと**掃除をしている）

Medical Terminology

Celsius	摂氏（℃）	health insurance card	健康保険証
Employees' Health Insurance	健康保険	National Health Insurance	国民健康保険
Fahrenheit	華氏（℉）	reference	紹介状
general hospital	総合病院	sluggish	不調の

Japanese Health Insurance（日本の健康保険）

　健（32歳）の妻のスーザン（30歳）はアメリカ人で，この春から日本での生活を始めましたが，まだ日本の生活に慣れていません。日本語の問題もあり，最近あまり夜，寝ることができず，さらに微熱が続いています。

▶ 体温の表し方を覚えましょう。
▶ 日本の医療システムはどのようになっているのでしょう。
▶ 日本の医療保険について確認しましょう。

Ken: Good morning, Susan. Has your fever gone down already?

Susan: Good morning, Ken. I feel sluggish with a slight fever. It was 99 degrees Fahrenheit.

What does Fahrenheit mean?

It is a scale of temperature usually used in the US. 99 degrees Fahrenheit is about 37 degrees Celsius. I have had a slight fever for some time.

That's not good and you had better go to hospital today. I will ask Mariko to take care of Taro.

Thank you. I will go to hospital in the morning, but I have never been to hospital to be examined in Japan. Do you have a family doctor near here?

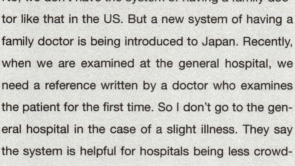 No, we don't have the system of having a family doctor like that in the US. But a new system of having a family doctor is being introduced to Japan. Recently, when we are examined at the general hospital, we need a reference written by a doctor who examines the patient for the first time. So I don't go to the general hospital in the case of a slight illness. They say the system is helpful for hospitals being less crowded.

Then taking your advice, I will go to the hospital.

That sounds good. Don't forget to take the health insurance card.

Is that insurance card a private health insurance card?

No, it isn't. It isn't a private insurance card. There are two principal types of insurance programs in Japan. One type is Kokumin-Kenko-Hoken.

What does Kokumin-Kenko-Hoken mean?

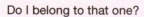 It means National Health Insurance.

Do I belong to that one?

No. This is for people who do not belong to any employment-based health insurance programs.

I am not employed.

The family members of employees are also involved in the Employees' Health Insurance or so called Kenko-Hoken, which is the other type of insurance program. This is for people employed at companies, schools and other occupational groups. Japanese residents should be enrolled in either National Health Insurance or Employees' Health Insurance. When insured people are examined or given medicine at hospitals or clinics, they have only to pay a part of the cost. I will pay 30% of the amount, the remaining of which the National Health Insurance Federation pays to medical facilities.

The Japanese insurance system is for all people living in Japan, isn't it? This program is wonderful and so Japanese average life span is much longer than that of other countries, I believe.

Maybe so, but there are big problems about National Health Insurance program. Japanese society is aging very rapidly, which causes much more medical expense. We are so worried that we won't be able to use medical facilities cheaply in the future.

Both Japan and the US have the difficulties regarding medical insurance system and medical treatment cost.

Anyway, you must take Employees' Health Insurance card of our family today. You are registered in the card.

I will go to hospital with the card.

Additional Medical Expressions

(4) I have never been to hospital to be examined.
診察で病院に行ったことがありません。

現在完了形の経験を表します。be examined は「診察してもらう」。

(5) We need a reference written by a doctor.
医師に書いてもらった紹介状が必要です。

reference の動詞は refer（紹介する）。〔The patient was referred to this hospital by A doctor.〕

(6) Don't forget to take the health insurance card.
健康保険証を持っていくのを忘れてはいけません。

forget to ～ は「これからすることを忘れる」。forget ～ ing は「**すでにしたことを忘れる**」。〔I forgot promising to meet him. 彼に会うと約束したことを忘れた。〕

Let's Use Communication Strategies！

相手の使った語・句が理解できず，聞き返すＣＳ

　相手が話した語句を理解できないことがよくあると思います。そのようなときに聞き返す方法を次の例で見てみましょう。

例1）p.3-l.11

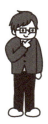
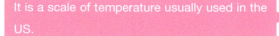
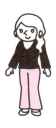

It was 99 degrees Fahrenheit.

What does Fahrenheit mean?

It is a scale of temperature usually used in the US.

例2）p.4-l.17

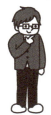
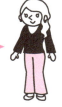

One type is Kokumin-Kenko-Hoken.

What does Kokumin-Kenko-Hoken mean?

It means National Health Insurance.

　医療従事者は患者，患者の家族，他の医療従事者からの情報・指示等を正しく聞き取ることが必要です。理解できない単語や語句があったら聞き直して正しい情報・指示等を得るようにしましょう。

Medical Sheet（問診表）

　診察前に患者が問診表に記入することで，自分の症状や病歴などを明確にでき，診察時間を有効に使えます。問診表の種類や内容はさまざまですが，次に内科の問診表の一例を挙げてあります。問診表に限らず，氏名，生年月日，性別などは記入する機会があると思いますので書き方に慣れておきましょう。

　受診の理由や病歴は一般的な症状や疾患名を覚えるよい機会になると思います。一度に専門英語語彙を覚えるのは難しいでしょうが，少しずつ覚えていきましょう。

Medical Terminology

abdominal pain	腹痛
allergic	アレルギーの
asthma	喘息
blood transfusion	輸血
bloody stool	血便
breast-feed	母乳で育てる
chest pain	胸痛
chill	寒気
constipation	便秘
diabetes	糖尿病
diarrhea	下痢
dizziness	めまい
fatigue	倦怠
feel weak	だるい
general physical weariness	全身倦怠感
high blood pressure	高血圧
hypertension	高血圧
internal medicine	内科
joint pain	関節痛
kidney	腎臓
letter of referral	紹介状
liver	肝臓
medical sheet	問診表（または medical questionnaire）
menopause	更年期
nausea	吐き気
numbness	しびれ
outpatient	外来患者
palpitation	動悸
period	月経期間
phlegm	痰
pneumonia	肺炎
poor appetite	食欲不振
prescribe	処方する
rash	発疹
shortness of breath	息切れ
sore throat	咽頭痛
stroke	卒中
symptom	症状
tuberculosis	結核
urination	排尿
vomiting	嘔吐

Medical Sheet for Outpatients (Internal Medicine Department) *Check ✓ in the ☐ for corresponding items and fill in the ( ).*			
last name ( ), first name ( )		sex	☐ male ☐ female
date of birth	year ( )/month ( )/day ( )	age	

What are your symptoms?   ☐ fever (°C)   ☐ sore throat   ☐ constipation   ☐ cough   ☐ headache   ☐ vomiting   ☐ nausea   ☐ stomachache   ☐ abdominal pain   ☐ diarrhea   ☐ bloody stool   ☐ poor appetite   ☐ shortness of breath   ☐ chest pain   ☐ palpitation   ☐ numbness   ☐ high blood pressure   ☐ dizziness   ☐ fatigue   ☐ rash   ☐ abnormal urination   ☐ chill   ☐ others (   )   How long have you had the problem? (   )
Previous illness and the approximate age of the onset   ☐ hypertension   (years old)   ☐ pneumonia   (years old)   ☐ diabetes   (years old)   ☐ liver disease   (years old)   ☐ asthma   (years old)   ☐ kidney disease   (years old)   ☐ heart disease   (years old)   ☐ stroke   (years old)   ☐ cancer   (years old)   ☐ tuberculosis   (years old)   ☐ other disease: the name of the disease (   ) (years old)
Have you had surgery?   ☐ no   ☐ yes (years old)
Have you had a blood transfusion?   ☐ no   ☐ yes (years old)
Do you have a food allergy?   ☐ no   ☐ yes (name of the food:)
Are you allergic to any medication?   ☐ no   ☐ yes (name of the medicine:)
Are you currently under medical treatment?   ☐ no   ☐ yes
Are you currently taking medicine?   ☐ no   ☐ yes (name of the medicine:)
Do you smoke?   ☐ no   ☐ yes but quit (   ) years ago.   ☐ yes (cigarettes/day)

Do you drink?   ☐ no   ☐ yes but quit (   ) years ago
         ☐ yes (type of alcohol: ☐ beer ☐ wine ☐ liquor ☐ others (   ))
              (frequency: ☐ almost everyday
                           ☐ a few times/week
                           ☐ a few times/month)

Questions for women   Are you pregnant?   ☐ no   ☐ not sure   ☐ yes (weeks)   Are you currently breast-feeding your baby?   ☐ no   ☐ yes   When was your last period?   (month/day: /)   Are you post menopausal?   ☐ no   ☐ yes
Do you have a letter of referral or the results of a medical examination?   ☐ no ☐ yes
Do you object to the use of generic medicine in your treatment?   ☐ no ☐ yes

Helpful English Grammar

1. They say 〜：〜らしい，〜といわれている

They say the system is helpful for the hospital being less crowded.
そのシステムは病院が混雑しないように役立っている**らしい**。

・**They say 〜** の英文を受動態に変えると，**It is said 〜** となります。

They say my mother was so cute when she was young.
→ It is said my mother was so cute when she was young.

2. 現在完了：have ＋ 過去分詞

過去から現在までの動作の完了，経験，継続を表します。

Has your fever gone down already?
もう熱は下がりましたか？〔完了を表す〕

I have never been to hospital.
病院に行ったことがありません。〔今までの経験を表す〕

3. The former … , the latter 〜：前者は…で，後者は〜です。

The former is for people who don't belong to any employment-based health insurance programs and **the latter** is for people employed at companies, schools, and other occupational groups.
前者はどの健康保険制度にも所属していない人のためのもので，**後者は**会社，学校，その他の職業グループに雇用されている人のためのものです。

4. 指示代名詞の that

文中ですでに述べられた名詞を指します。

Japanese average life span is much longer than **that of** other countries.
日本人の平均寿命は他の国よりずっと長い。

・that は average life span を示しています。

A drinker's brain is smaller than **that of** a nondrinker.
　飲酒者の脳は非飲酒者の脳より小さい。

・**複数形の場合は those となります。**

Mariko's eyes are bigger than **those** of Ken.
　真理子の目は健の目より大きい。

ほっと一息!

アメリカの医療保険

　アメリカには日本のような国民皆保険制度がありません。そのため，国民の大多数は雇用先が提供する医療保険や個人で加入する民間保険に加入しています。しかし，2009 年時点においては 5070 万人以上が無保険者であり，政府はこれらの人々のために以下の公的医療保険制度を設けています。

65 歳以上の高齢者や障害者を対象としたメディケア

　1965 年に設立され，社会保障法（Social Security Act）第 18 章に規定されています。1973 年には，高齢者のみならず，障害者や腎臓移植や人工透析が必要な末期腎臓病患者にも適用されるようになりました。

貧困者を対象としたメディケイド

　1965 年に設立され，はじめは母子家庭を救済する目的でしたが，貧困者の救済に適用されるようになりました。

18 歳以下の児童を対象とした児童保険プログラム制度

　1997 に設立された低所得者世帯の無保険児のための保険で，2009 年にはこの保険を改善延長する児童医療保険プログラム再認可法が成立しました。

　2010 年 3 月に，オバマ大統領の署名により医療制度改革法が成立し，国民皆保険導入の実現への動きが始まっています。

Chapter 2
Internal Medicine: Influenza
内科：インフルエンザ

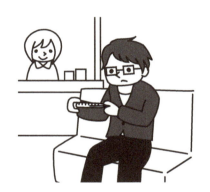

　熱があり，咳などの症状で病院を受診した時の，インフルエンザ特有の症状，検査，治療方法を会話で学びましょう。

　インフルエンザはインフルエンザウイルスにより発生します。インフルエンザを発症した場合は迅速に治療することが重要です。重症化すると肺炎になる可能性があるため，幼児，高齢者は特に注意をする必要があります。

Purposes of this Chapter

臨床英語表現	インフルエンザの症状・治療に関連する表現
コミュニケーション・ストラテジー	相手の発言を受け止めていることを知らせる
医療従事者の知識	インフルエンザについての正しい知識
重要構文	not only … but also，分詞の後置修飾

Medical Dialogue

Basic Medical Expressions

医療現場でよく使われる簡単な表現です。自然に言えるようになるまで声に出して何度も読み，完全に覚えましょう。

---

7 Do you have a sore throat?
のどの痛みはありますか？

症状の有無を尋ねるのに Do you have …? をよく使います。

---

8 The coughing started this morning.
今朝から咳がでます。

症状の始まった時期を start を使って表せます。

---

9 I hope you get well soon.
早く良くなるといいですね。

「お大事に」と言いたいときにもよく使います。

---

10 It will take about 15 minutes to have the result.
検査結果がでるのに 15 分かかります。

「時間がかかる」は It takes …，「結果がでる」は have が使えます。

Medical Terminology

〜 degrees Celsius	摂氏〜℃	inhalation	吸入
antipyretic	解熱剤	muscle pain	筋肉痛
antiviral drug	抗ウイルス薬	nasal discharge	鼻水
chilly	寒さでぞくぞくする	swab	綿棒
diagnose	診断する	tablet	錠剤
dose	1回服用量	uncomfortable	不快な
general fatigue	全身倦怠感	virus	ウイルス
influenza	インフルエンザ		

Internal Medicine（内科）

　前夜からの発熱と頭痛が朝になっても良くなっていない健（32歳）は、内科を受診することにしました。待合室で体温を測り、問診表の記入も済ませ、診察室で医師の診察を受けています。

▶ 健にはどのような症状があるのでしょう。
▶ インフルエンザ検査はどのようにするのでしょう。
▶ インフルエンザ治療はどのようにされるのでしょう。

In the internal medicine department:

Ken

Good morning, Doctor.

Doctor

Morning, Mr. Kato. I've heard you have a high fever. When did you notice it?

After I ate dinner last night, I felt chilly and had a headache. Later I took my temperature … I think it was at about nine.

Okay. Do you remember your temperature then?

It was the same as it is now.

I see. It is 38.6 degrees Celsius now.

That's right.

Do you have a sore throat, joint pain or a cough?

Yes. I have a terrible headache and a sore throat. The coughing started this morning with yellowish phlegm.

 I see. How about muscle pain or joint pain?

 I have muscle pain in my arms and legs. I don't have joint pain but I feel really weak.

 I see. So you have general fatigue. Do you have nausea, stomachache, or diarrhea?

 No, I don't.

 Does anyone in your family have similar symptoms?

 Not in my family but some people absent from my workplace have similar symptoms.

 Oh, really? You may have influenza. We will need to test to properly diagnose. I will put a swab in your nose and sample your nasal discharge for testing. It may be uncomfortable but please be patient.

 Okay.

 That's it. It will take about 15 minutes to have the results. Please wait in the waiting room and we'll call you when the results are ready.

About 15 minutes later:

> The result has come from the laboratory. It is positive for the influenza A type virus. I will prescribe an antiviral drug so that the condition will not get worse. The effects will last for about 5 days for each dose by inhalation. It will take a day or two to lower your temperature, and you can take antipyretic tablets for your high fever. You can take two tablets when your fever is higher than 38 degrees Celsius. But you must not take another dose for another six hours. You should feel better in five or six days. If you experience severe dizziness, please let us know immediately. Do you have any questions?

> No. Thank you very much.

> I hope you get well soon.

Additional Medical Expressions

11 It may be uncomfortable but please be patient.
少し嫌な感じがするかもしれませんが，我慢してくださいね。
un- をつければ comfortable の反意語ですね。

12 You can take two tablets when your fever is higher than 38 degrees Celsius.
熱が 38℃以上のときには 2 錠飲んでいいですよ。
「薬を飲む」のに drink は使いません。温度に華氏 Fahrenheit を使う場合もあります。

(13) You must not take another dose for another six hours.
次の服用まで6時間は間を空けてください。

another の使い方に慣れましょう。

(14) If you experience severe dizziness, please let me know immediately.
もしひどいめまいがあったら，すぐにお知らせください。

症状があることを「経験する（experience）」でも表現できます。「させて」という用法の let もよく使います。

Let's Use Communication Strategies！

相手の発言を受け止めていることを知らせる CS

I see.（p.14-l.16, p.15-l.4, 7）; Okay.（p.14-l.14, p.15-l.18）; Oh really?（p.15-l.14）

　これらがなくても会話で伝える内容に違いはなさそうですが，会話の雰囲気がずいぶんと違ってきます。CS の有無による違いを感じましょう。

 I took my temperature … I think it was at about nine.

Okay. Do you remember your temperature then?

　「言ったことをちゃんと聞いてもらえてるな…よかった！」と感じますね。この "Okay." がないと「こちらの答えにおかまいなしで次の質問って感じで，ちょっとさみしい！」と感じますね。

 It was the same as it is now.

> I see. It is 38.6 degrees Celsius now.

"I see." があると「はっきり数字を言えなかったけど，わかってもらえてよかった！」という感じになりますね。"I see." がないと「数字を言えなくて叱られているみたいでみじめ…」と感じませんか？

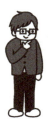

> Not in my family but some people are absent from my workplace because of the similar symptoms.

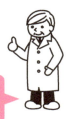

> Oh, really? You may have influenza and we need to examine to diagnose.

"Oh, really?" と言ってくれたことで，「余分なことかと思ったけど，同僚のことも言ってよかったんだ！」もし，"Oh, really?" がないと，「こっちの言ったこと参考にならなかったのかな？　余分なこと言っちゃったのか」と心配になりますね。

　これらの CS は，相手の言ったことに対して「ちゃんと聞いてるよ」「わかるよ」というメッセージを送ることになります。お互いにより気持ちよく話せるようにこうした CS をどんどん使いましょう。

B　Medical Reading

Medical Terminology

acetaminophen	アセトアミノフェン（解熱鎮痛剤）	cervix	くび，頚部
antibody	抗体	contraindicate	（薬・療法など）に禁忌を示す

encephalopathy	脳症（脳疾患）	reddened	赤くなった
epidemic	伝染病，流行	shivering	悪寒戦慄
fever convulsion	熱性痙攣	swollen	腫れ上がった（swell の過去分詞形）
immunity	免疫（性）		
Inavir Dry Powder Inhaler	イナビル吸入剤	Tamiflu capsule	タミフルカプセル剤
pharynx	咽頭		

Influenza（インフルエンザ）

　　Influenza is an infectious disease caused by influenza viruses. It is also known as "the flu" by many people. Not only influenza virus A but also influenza virus B spreads in seasonal epidemics, especially in winter.

　　During influenza seasonal epidemics, a person with some mixtures of symptoms such as a high fever, chills, shivering, a cough, a headache, body aches（especially joints and throat）, fatigue and reddened eyes and face can be identified as one infected with the influenza virus. Some symptoms occur suddenly after the infection. Infants and babies suffering from influenza sometimes have a high fever（over 39℃）, fever convulsions, and a swollen cervix lymph. We should especially watch for encephalopathy in children under 5 with a high fever（over 39℃）.

　　To distinguish between the common cold and influenza is sometimes difficult, but influenza can be diagnosed in 15 minutes by testing a nasal drop of liquid from the pharynx. The rapidness of the test makes it easier to decide whether the patient has influenza or not.

　　As soon as the influenza virus is found, it is important to take effective preventative measures so as not to transmit the influenza virus to another person. Particularly it is essential to prevent the virus from infecting infants, old people, and the patients with less immunity.

Moreover, patients with influenza may develop pneumonia.

The treatment against influenza is taking antiviral drugs. Within 48 hours after being infected by the influenza virus, two antiviral drugs, the use of Tamiflu capsule or an Inavir Dry Powder Inhaler is common. For children under 5 years old, the use of Tamiflu capsule is contraindicated because of the reports the medicine can cause young children to behave abnormally. For patients with a high fever, acetaminophen is prescribed.

Nowadays the news that a new influenza virus which is tolerant of the Tamiflu capsule has appeared and human beings were infected with bird influenza has been reported, which is both surprising and worrisome to us.

Comprehension

1) 本文の内容について，次の問いに英語で答えなさい。

1. What causes influenza?
2. What are symptoms of influenza?
3. How long does it take to get the result of influenza?
4. What medicine is prescribed for influenza within 48 hours?
5. What surprises and worries us about influenza recently?

2) 本文の内容に合うように語群より適切な語句を選び，(　　) に入れなさい。

The influenza is known as (1), which is transmitted widely by (2), sneezing, touching (3) and eating infected food. When you get influenza, you will have some symptoms such as a high fever, a (4), (5), body ache and so on. You should go to hospital, and after (6) as influenza, you should take a rest and take medicine. The most important thing is not to transmit influenza virus to another person.

headache	coughing	heavy	fatigue
flu	nasal secretion	being diagnosed	

Helpful English Grammar

1. not only A but (also) B：A ばかりではなく B も

Not only influenza virus A but also influenza virus B spreads in seasonal epidemics, especially in winter.

　インフルエンザ A 型だけでなく B 型も季節の流行で広まります。特に冬に広まります。

・not only A but also B は B as well as A と同じ意味を表します。

2. 分詞の後置修飾

Infants and babies suffering from influenza sometimes have a high fever (over 39℃), a headache, coughing and heavy fatigue.

　インフルエンザで苦しんでいる幼児や赤ん坊には時々高熱，頭痛，咳，ひどい倦怠感があります。

・分詞の後に目的語や修飾語句がついて**分詞句**になると後ろから前の名詞を修飾します。

・**現在分詞（～ ing）は「～する，～している」，過去分詞は「～されている，～された」**の意味で名詞を修飾します。

(例)

Who is the girl **playing the piano** over there?

　ピアノを弾いている少女

My friend is always reading books **written in English**.

　英語で書かれた本

ほっと一息！

Q インフルエンザ予防方法として「部屋の中でぬれタオルを振りまわすのが一番！」って時々いわれますが，これは本当かな〜？

A インフルエンザ予防として湿度管理が重要です。室内の湿度は50%〜60%を保つことが効果的です。室内でぬれタオルや加湿器を使用するのがいいといわれています。室内にぬれタオルを置くだけよりも振りまわしたほうが湿度が上がると考えたのでしょう。湿度保持のためには効果があります。

厚労省が出しているインフルエンザ対策を紹介いたします。
1. 流行前のワクチン接種
2. 飛沫感染対策としてマスク使用
3. 外出後の手洗い
4. 適切な湿度維持
5. 十分な休養とバランスの取れた栄養摂取
6. 人ごみや繁華街への外出を控える

特に手洗いは流水で手の指一本一本を丁寧に洗うことが重要です。この簡単な手洗いが病気予防の第一歩です。

Let's wash our hands carefully !

Chapter 3
Nurse
看護師

外国人が初めて日本のクリニックを訪れた時の様子を会話例で学びましょう。

看護師はあらゆる年齢層の人たちの健康促進，疾病予防，健康回復，痛みの緩和など幅広い役割を担っています。看護師の役割と歴史について学びましょう。

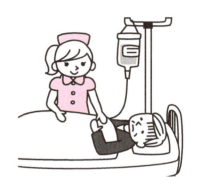

Purposes of this Chapter

臨床英語表現	体調不良の症状に関する表現
コミュニケーション・ストラテジー	相手の会話を受け入れて，会話を進める
医療従事者の知識	体調不良と看護師についての正しい知識
重要構文	比較級＋比較級，so as to 〜 = in order to, despite = in spite of, It is not until 〜 that …

Medical Dialogue

Basic Medical Expressions

医療現場でよく使われる簡単な表現です。自然に言えるようになるまで声に出して何度も読み，完全に覚えましょう。

15 Is this your first time visiting us?
今回が初めてのご来院ですか？

16 Do you have your appointment with us today?
今日は予約されていますか？

17 What brought you here today?
今日はどうされましたか？
what が主語。

Medical Terminology

armpit	腋下	sleep disorder	睡眠障害
mother-in-law	義理の母	thermometer	体温計

First Visit to a Clinic（クリニックへの最初の訪問）

　スーザン（30歳）は日本での生活に慣れないためか，体調不良が続いています。義理の母親の真理子（60歳）に息子の太郎（5歳）を預けて，近所のクリニックに来ています。

▷ 誰がクリニックに予約したのでしょう。
▷ 受付ではじめに何をするように言われたのでしょう。
▷ 体温計の使い方をどのように指示されたのでしょう。

At the information desk in a clinic:

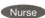
Nurse: Hello, is this your first time visiting us?

Susan: Oh yes, this is the first time for me.

Do you have an appointment with us today?

Yes, mother-in-law, Mariko called instead of me.

OK. I will check the appointment sheet. Are you Susan Kato?

Yes, I am.

What brought you here today?

I have been tired with a slight fever for a few days and have a sleep disorder.

That's too bad. First of all, would you fill in this medical sheet while you are waiting to be called?

Maybe I can't do because I cannot read Japanese.

Don't worry. This medical sheet is written in English.

Oh, really? I feel at ease to hear that.

There are so many foreign people in this area that we prepare an English medical sheet and all our medical staff can understand English.

Really? I didn't know that.

Here you are. Please fill in this sheet in detail in order for the doctor to understand your condition.

I see.

Susan is filling in the medical sheet:

I have finished doing it.

 Please take your temperature with this clinical thermometer, placing it under your armpit for a few minutes.

My body temperature was 37°C.

 OK. Please be seated until the doctor calls you into the room.

Additional Medical Expressions

(18) Please fill in this medical sheet while you are waiting to be called.
お待ちになっている間にこの問診表に記入してください。

(19) Please take your temperature with this clinical thermometer placing it under your armpit.
体温計を脇の下に入れて体温を測ってください。
「脇の下」ではなく「舌の下」では under your tongue になります。

(20) Please be seated until the doctor calls you into the room.
名前が呼ばれるまでお座りください。

Let's Use Communication Strategies！

相手の発言に簡単な反応を示す CS

　相手の話が同情すべき内容だった場合に「それはお気の毒です」「それはいけませんね」などという気持ちを伝える "That's too bad." と相手の話の内容について知らなかった場合，新情報を聞いたときの「それは，知りませんでした」と，"I didn't know that." を使えるようになりましょう。

That's too bad. の例：p.25-l.12

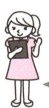
I have been tired with a slight fever for a few days and have a sleep disorder.

That's too bad. First of all, would you fill in this medical sheet ….
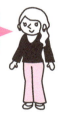

　スーザンの訴えを聞いた看護師が「それはいけませんね」と気持ちを伝えてから，問診表への記入を依頼しています。この一言があることで，スーザンは「自分の苦痛がわかってもらえた」と感じます。

I didn't know that. の例：p.25-l.20

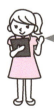
There are so many foreign people in this area that we prepare an English medical sheet and all our medical staff can understand English.

Really? I didn't know that.
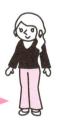

　看護師の言った内容をスーザンは「知らなかった」と伝えているだけのように聞こえますが，相手から提供された情報を知っているのか，知らなかったのかを伝えることは，その情報をきちんと受け止めていることを相手に示すこと

となります。新情報であれば、提供した相手も「知らせてあげてよかった」という満足感が得られることでしょう。

Medical Reading

Medical Terminology

acupuncturist	鍼灸師	pharmacist	薬剤師
beriberi	脚気	physical therapist	理学療法士
drug administration	与薬	public health nurse	保健師
International Council of Nurses（ICN）	国際看護師協会	radiologist	放射線技師
midwife	助産師	registered dietitian（RD）	管理栄養士
monastery	（主に男子の）修道院		

Nurse（看護師）

　A nurse has very wide roles such as taking care of many kinds of patients, diseases, people from different age groups and promoting their lives. A report from the International Council of Nurses shows that nurses have four responsibilities to accomplish their duties: promotion of health, prevention of disease, restoring of health, and relief of pain. Under the guidance of doctors, they do their best to carry out their duties. They work to treat patients, drug administration, check patients' body conditions and so on. Nowadays their work is getting wider and wider because of increased chronic diseases, more aged people and more variety of diseases. Moreover they have to work with not only doctors but many other medical staff (pharmacists, registered dietitians, physical therapists, radiologists, acupuncturists, etc.). Through their daily work, they build up their careers and keep studying in order to do very special care as qualified nurses. Some nurses become public health nurses or midwives.

The history of nurses began in ancient churches. People living in churches had been taking care of the disordered or sick people and the dying. A leader of the church, St. Benedict of Nursia who built a monastery advocated the importance of medicine. In the middle age, monks and sisters in the Catholic Church built charity facilities to care for old people, orphans and sick persons as nurses. In the nineteenth century, a nurse named Florence Nightingale looked after lots of the wounded and the dying in the Crimean War and established the base of nurse education, which has developed through years.

In Japan some training schools of nurses were founded and influenced by the idea of Florence Nightingale. Kanehiro Takagi, a well-known person, who conducted research into beriberi, founded the first training school in 1885, because he recognized the importance of nurses' professions while studying in the U.K. Despite his efforts, most nurses got medical knowledge through practical works without studying in the training school he founded.

After World War II, Japanese nurses' education has been much reformed by the influence of American nurses' education. A student who wanted to be a nurse began to learn at university or a training school of nurses to get medical knowledge.

The persons working as nurses were all women before, but recently more and more men have begun to work as nurses, and so it was not until 2002 that the called name was unified to "kangoshi (看護師)". That is to say, before 2002 the called name and Chinese letter of "kangoshi" were different: "kangofu (看護婦)" for women and "kangoshi (看護士)" for men.

    Today more and more nurses are needed in accordance with treating increased chronic diseases and more aged people and managing advanced medical equipment. This circumstance makes it necessary that they get much more medical knowledge and do special technology focused in advanced medicine. The number of students studying at university to be a nurse is increasing more and more in Japan. Japanese nurses with much skillful medical knowledge and careers will be able to treat patients independently like special nurses in the US in the future.

Comprehension

1）本文の内容について，次の問いに英語で答えなさい。

1. What does a report from the International Council of Nurses show?
2. What did St. Benedict of Nursia do?
3. What did Kanehiro Takagi do?
4. When was the called name of a nurse changed in Japan?
5. What kinds of things are requested of a nurse recently?

2）次の文を英文に訳しなさい。

1. 仙台に住んでいる私の従兄は看護師です。
2. 看護師は毎日忙しく患者の世話をしている。
3. 私の叔母は今病院に入院しています。病院では看護師さんによく世話をしてもらっています。

Helpful English Grammar

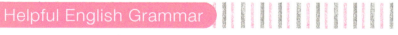

1. wider and wider：比較級＋比較級：ますます〜，だんだん〜

Nowadays their work is **getting wider and wider** because of increased chronic diseases, more aged people and more variety of diseases.

今日，慢性疾患の増加，高齢者の増加，さまざまの疾患のために，彼らの仕**事はますます広がっています。**

・不規則な比較級を覚えましょう！

good - better, bad - worse, many - more, little - less

比較級で語尾変化をしない語彙は **more and more** を前につけます。

Flowers are getting **more and more beautiful** in spring.

花は春にますます綺麗になります。

2. so as to 〜 = in order to 〜：〜するために

They build up their careers and keep studying **so as to** do very special care as a qualified nurse.

彼らは資格を得た看護師として**特別な介護をするために**キャリアを積み，勉強を続けています。

・to 以下を否定する時は to の前に not を入れます。

They study medicine **so as not to** make medical errors.

医療過誤をしないために彼らは医学を勉強します。

3. despite = in spite of：〜にもかかわらず

despite his efforts

彼の努力にも**かかわらず**

4. It was not until 〜 that …：〜して初めて（やっと）…した

It **was not until** 2003 **that** the called name was unified to "kangoshi (*看護師*)".

2003 年になって初めて，呼び名が看護師に統一された。

・この英文は It is 〜 that の強調構文です。

It was not until yesterday that I could finish my report.

昨日になってやっとレポートを終えることできた。

日本の看護師制度

　日本における看護師の免許には「看護師」と「准看護師」があり，看護師は大学，短大，専門学校で合計3000時間以上の養成教育がなされます。修了後に国家試験を受け，合格者には厚生労働大臣から看護師免許が交付され看護師として活動できるようになります。「准看護師」は准看護師学校，看護系の高等学校で1890時間以上の教育を受け終了後，都道府県知事試験を受け，合格者には都道府県知事から准看護師の免許が交付されます。看護師に益々高度な知識が要求される昨今，准看護師の廃止の動きもあります。

　以下はアメリカの上級看護師であるナースプラクティショナーについての英文です。トライしてみましょう。

　In the US, there are different kinds of nurses, who are called "nurse practitioners". A Nurse Practitioner is a profession with special knowledge for treating diseases. They can do the same kinds of work as those of physicians and physician assistants, which means they can prescribe and treat patients without the guidance of doctors. Most of these nurses graduated from postgraduate school and received a master's degree. They work at hospital for doing primary care. This system is not in Japan.

Chapter 4
Internal Medicine: Hepatic Disease
内科：肝炎

体調不良のため病院に行った時，医者はどのような質問を患者にするのかを会話例で学びましょう。

急性肝炎は肝臓疾患の一つで，主な原因はA，B，およびC型肝炎ウイルスによるものです。発熱，全身倦怠，食欲不振などの症状があり，十分な休息を取ることが必要です。

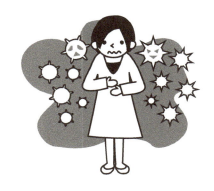

Purposes of this Chapter

臨床英語表現	急性肝炎の症状・治療に関する表現
コミュニケーション・ストラテジー	相手の言ったことが理解できないときに聞き直す
医療従事者の知識	肝炎についての正しい知識
重要構文	be likely to 〜，It 〜 that 〜の構文，generally speaking, judging from の分詞の慣用表現，It 〜 to 〜の構文（仮主語について）

A Medical Dialogue

Basic Medical Expressions

医療現場でよく使われる簡単な表現です。自然に言えるようになるまで声に出して何度も読み，完全に覚えましょう。

21
I have no appetite.
食欲がありません。

22
I don't have diarrhea but have a little nausea.
下痢はありませんが吐き気が少しあります。
「下痢」は略式で the runs，「吐き気」は sickness でもよい。「吐く，嘔吐する」は vomit。

23
I would like to run some blood tests.
血液検査をします。
「(実験などを) 行う」は run を使い，「run a check」で「検査をする」となります。run には「(水・涙・鼻水などを) 流す」という意味もあります。(My nose is running.(鼻水が流れる))

Medical Terminology

acute appendicitis	急性虫垂炎	blood test	血液検査
acute hepatic disease	急性肝炎	diagnosis	診断
appetite	食欲		

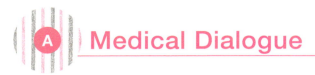
Internal Medicine（内科）

最近，加藤一郎（65歳）は庭の手入れをしているとすぐに疲れ，横になってしまいます。この状態が1か月ほど続くため，近所の内科医院で診察してもらうことにしました。内科医院の受付で簡単な問診を受け，診察室で医師の診察

を受けています。

▋▷ 一郎にはどのような症状があるのでしょう。

▋▷ 医師はどのような質問を一郎にしているのでしょう。

In the Consulting Room:

Doctor

What brought you in today?

I have been tired for a few days and the color of my urine was brown today. So I came here to be examined.

Ichiro

Do you have a fever?

My temperature was 37.6°C this morning, moreover I had no appetite.

Do you have nausea now? Did you have diarrhea or feel diarrhea?

I don't have diarrhea but have a little nausea.

Have you had a blood transfusion or an operation?

Pardon me?

I asked if you had had a blood transfusion or an operation.

Oh, I had an operation for an acute appendicitis when I was 19 years old but I didn't have a blood transfusion.

Do any of your family members have liver disease?

Nobody has liver disease in my family.

 Have you eaten raw oysters or seashells recently?

Would you say that again?

 Okay. Have you eaten raw oysters or seashells recently?

Oh! I traveled about a month ago and I ate a lot of raw oysters and seashells.

 I see. Mr. Kato, I would like to run some blood tests now.

Is my condition so bad?

 Don't worry. I will diagnose after I see the result.

 Mr. Kato, I will take you to the room for a clinical examination.

Thank you.

The result of the clinical examination was that Mr. Kato's liver was infected by a virus and the doctor's diagnosis for Mr. Kato was acute hepatic disease.

Additional Medical Expressions

24 Have you had a blood transfusion?
輸血を受けたことがありますか。

「輸血を受ける」は have / get / receive a blood transfusion と表現します。「輸血をする」は transfuse 〜 です。

25 I had an operation for an acute appendicitis.
急性虫垂炎の手術を受けました。

「手術を受ける」は undergo an operation という言い方もあります。

26 I will take you to the room for a clinical examination.
検査室にご案内します。

27 Positive rate for HAV antibody is about 90%.
HAV 抗体の陽性率は 90％です。

positive は検査結果でよく使います。「陰性」は negative です。

Let's Use Communication Strategies！

相手が言ったことが理解できないときに聞き直す CS

　会話で相手が言ったことが理解できないとき，そのままわかったふりをしていると困ることもあります。

昨日，佐藤君から電話があったのよ。

あ，そう…。

誰から電話があったって言ったのかしら？　聞こえなかったけど。

今度，一緒に遊びに来いって言ってたわよ。

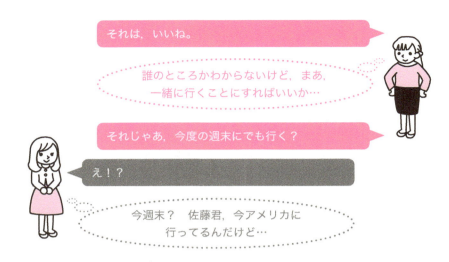

理解できないときは，次の例のように "Pardon me?" "Excuse me?" "Would you say that again?" などの表現で聞き返しましょう。

Pardon me?「え？ 何て言ったの？」の例：p.35-l.16

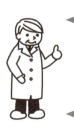
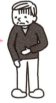

Have you had a blood transfusion or an operation?

Pardon me?

I asked if you had had a blood transfusion or an operation.

Would you say that again?「もう一度言ってください」の例：p.36-l.4

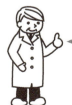
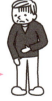

Have you eaten raw oysters or seashells recently?

Would you say that again?

Okay. Have you eaten raw oysters or seashells recently?

B Medical Reading

Medical Terminology

acute viral hepatitis	急性ウイルス性肝炎	hepatitis A virus	A型肝炎ウイルス
alcoholic liver disease	アルコール性肝炎	incubation period	潜伏期間
		inflammation	炎症
bile	胆汁	intestinal tract	腸管
contaminated water	汚染水	jaundice	黄疸
		manifestation	発症
fatty liver disease	脂肪肝	positive rate	陽性率
feces	便	prognosis	予後
fulminant hepatitis (FH)	劇症肝炎	triglyceride	中性脂肪
		vaccination	予防接種

〔肝臓の検査〕
・GOT：glutamic oxaloacetic transaminase　グルタミン酸オキサロ酢酸トランスアミナーゼ
・GPT：glutamic pyruvic transaminase　グルタミン酸ピルビン酸トランスアミナーゼ

　これらの酵素は細胞質に存在し，細胞が障害を受けると血液中に逸脱します。したがって，細胞障害の程度を表す指標として用いられます。GOTは肝細胞のほか，心筋，骨格筋にも含まれ，これらの組織が障害されると血中

濃度は高くなります。それに対し，GPTは主に肝細胞からの逸脱により血中濃度が上昇するため，肝障害の程度を把握するのに有用であり，より肝特異的です。

・γ-GTP：γ-glutamyl transpeptidase　γグルタミルトランスペプチダーゼ

　肝臓では毛細胆管に分布し，一部が血中に移行します。アルコール性肝障害，薬物性肝障害，慢性肝疾患，胆管がんなどで上昇し，肝細胞障害そのものよりも胆道系障害や胆汁うっ滞の指標として用いられます。

Acute Viral Hepatitis（AVH：急性ウイルス性肝炎）

Acute viral hepatitis is one of many kinds of liver diseases: for example there are alcoholic liver disease which is hepatic manifestation caused by alcohol overconsumption and fatty liver disease caused by accumulation of triglyceride because of taking much fats and sugar in liver cells and so on.

Hepatitis, inflammation of the liver is caused by many viruses, and acute viral hepatitis is focused on in this chapter.

The main causes of acute viral hepatitis are hepatitis A virus, hepatitis B virus and hepatitis C virus. Hepatitis A virus（HAV）is transmitted orally while hepatitis B virus as well as hepatitis C virus by blood. HAV increases in the hepatic cells and increased viruses are excreted into the intestinal tract through bile. Finally they are excreted with feces. In Japan it is reported a lot that HAV is spread by oral infection: eating raw oysters and seashells. In other countries, it was often spread by contaminated water and raw vegetables before.

In the Japanese, positive rate for HAV antibody is about 90% among adult over 60, while the positive rate in people under 40 is about 1%.

HAV is likely to spread from winter to the beginning of spring, especially in March and April.

The symptoms appear after an incubation period of two to six weeks: a fever, symptoms of cold, general fatigue, loss of appetite and nausea. In addition, the symptoms such as brown urine and jaundice sometimes appear.

Judging from the biochemistry test, the serum level of GOT, GPT and γ-GTP is increasing.

The treatment for the disease is taking a good rest and transfusion of sugar liquid. Generally speaking, the patient's prognosis is good but 1% of the patients develop the worst condition called fulminant hepatitis (FH). The most effective protection for HAV is vaccination. It is very important for people without antibody of HAV to get vaccination of HAV when traveling to Africa, Central Asia, Latin America and the South-East Asia.

Comprehension

1）本文の内容について，次の問いに英語で答えなさい。
1. What is the cause of fatty liver disease?
2. How are hepatitis A virus, B virus and C virus transmitted?
3. When is HAV likely to spread in Japan?
4. List the symptoms of HAV.
5. What is the worst condition of HAV?

2）本文の内容に合うように語群より適切な語句を選び，（　）に入れなさい。

Hepatitis is （ 1 ） of the liver. Both hepatitis B virus and hepatitis C virus are transmitted by （ 2 ）. Judging from the biochemistry test, the figures of （ 3 ）, GOT and γ-GTP get higher .

The treatment for the disease is taking a good rest and transfusion of

(4). The patient's prognosis is good but 1% of the patients goes to the worst condition called (5). The most effective protection for HAV is (6).

GPT	fulminant hepatitis	inflammation
hepatic A virus	vaccination　　blood	sugar liquid

Helpful English Grammar

1. be likely to ＋動詞の原型：〜する傾向にある

HAV **is likely to** spread from winter to the beginning of spring.

　HAV は冬から春の初めに広がる**傾向にある**。

He **is likely to** be elected president of the country.

　彼はその国の大統領に当選しそうだ。

・be likely to の反対は be **unlikely to** 〜で「〜しそうにない」

2. It ＋形容詞（名詞）that …

　It は形式主語で，that … が本主語です。

It is reported a lot **that HAV is spread by oral infection**.

　HAV は経口感染することが報告されている。

・It が形式主語で **to 以下が本主語**の例文は以下のものです。

It is very important **for people** without antibody of HAV **to get vaccination of HAV** in traveling to Africa, Central Asia, Latin America and the South-East Asia.

　HAV の抗体を持たない人がアフリカ，中央アジア，ラテンアメリカ，東南アジアを旅行する時，**HAV の予防接種をすること**がとても重要です。

・**for people** は to 以下の英文の行為者なので（**〜たちが…するのは…です**）と日本語にしたほうが理解しやすいです。

・to 〜 以下を否定するときは **to の前に not** を入れます。

It is good **not to eat too much**.

　食べ過ぎないことはいいことです。

3. 分詞の慣用表現

judging from 〜：〜から判断すると，generally speaking：一般的に言うと，considering 〜：〜を考慮に入れると，frankly speaking：率直に言って，talking of 〜：〜と言えば

ほっと一息！

ウイルス性肝炎の種類

肝炎の種類	原因肝炎ウイルス	発見年度
A型肝炎	A型肝炎ウイルス	1973年
B型肝炎	B型肝炎ウイルス	1964年
C型肝炎	C型肝炎ウイルス	1989年
D型肝炎	D型肝炎ウイルス	1977年
E型肝炎	E型肝炎ウイルス	1980年
F型肝炎	F型肝炎ウイルス	1994年

A型肝炎，B型肝炎，C型肝炎が多いです。

海外渡航のためのワクチン接種

　海外渡航のためのワクチン接種には，渡航する国からの予防接種証明要求に応じる目的と，自分または関係者への感染予防の目的があります。

- 南米の熱帯地域（中央アフリカ，中南米）では入国時に黄熱ワクチンの予防接種証明書の提示が求められます。入国の10日以上前にトラベルクリニックや検疫所で接種を受けましょう。
- 途上国に出かける場合，黄熱以外ではA型ワクチン接種が重要です。渡航先の感染の流行状態により，B型ワクチン，破傷風ワクチン，腸チフス，または狂犬病のワクチン接種を受けるようにしましょう。
- ワクチンにより接種回数が異なります。→黄熱ワクチン　　　1回
　　　　　　　　　　　　　　　　　　　　A型肝炎ワクチン　3回
　　　　　　　　　　　　　　　　　　　　破傷風トキソイド　3回
　　　　　　　　　　　　　　　　　　　　狂犬病ワクチン　　3回

Chapter 5

Blood Test: Medical Technologist

血液検査：臨床検査技師

採血は医師や看護師以外に臨床検査技師によって実施されることがあります。採血時には患者に説明や依頼をしたり，患者から情報を聞き取ったりしなければなりません。そのための英語表現を会話例で学びましょう。

臨床検査技師は血液の他に，どのような検体を採取して検査室で調べるのでしょうか。また，検体検査以外にも臨床検査技師が行う検査があります。読み取りましょう。

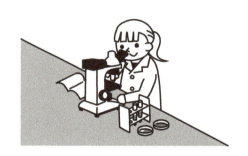

Purposes of this Chapter

臨床英語表現	血液検査や臨床検査技師に関連する表現
コミュニケーション・ストラテジー	相手の発言の一部分を聞き返す
医療従事者の知識	臨床検査技師の仕事
重要構文	of の用法，副詞の用法

Medical Dialogue

Basic Medical Expressions

　医療現場でよく使われる簡単な表現です。自然に言えるようになるまで声に出して何度も読み，完全に覚えましょう。

---

28 Can you take off your jacket?
上着を脱げますか。

Can you…？　と，疑問文の形ですが依頼の目的で使っています。

---

29 Let me rub your arm.
腕を拭きますね。

アルコール綿で拭く時も rub を使います。

---

30 Please make a fist with your thumb in.
親指を中に入れて握り拳をつくってください。

付帯状況の with です。

Medical Terminology

gauze	ガーゼ	sterile	無菌の
injection	注射	sting	痛む（チクチクした痛み）
medical technologist	臨床検査技師	vein	静脈
sample	検体		

Blood Test（血液検査）

　一郎（65 歳）は長期にわたる倦怠感，発熱，食欲不振等から内科を受診しています。肝臓疾患の疑いから血液検査を受けることになり，検査室の外で番号札をもって採血の順番を待っています（MT：medical technologist）。

▶ 一郎の採血はどのような職種の人によってなされたでしょう。

■▷ 採血に際し,一郎にどのような指示や質問がされたでしょう。
■▷ 採血はどのような手順でなされたでしょう。

 Does anyone have the number card two-one-four?

 The number two-one-what?

 Two-one-four.

 Thank you. I have the number.

 Would you come in this room?

 All right.

 Would you sit here? You can put your belongings in the basket there.

 Thank you.

 Would you tell me your full name and date of birth, please?

 I am Ichiro Kato. I was born on June 21st, 1949.

 Thank you. My name is Yokoi. I'm a medical technologist.

 You are a medical what?

 A medical technologist.

Oh, a medical technologist. Is it usual for a medical technologist to take a blood sample?

 Yes, especially in large hospitals.

 A nurse gives me injections at the clinic I usually go to for consultation.

 Medical technologists cannot give injections.

 Oh, really? They put in needles, when giving injections or taking blood samples.

 Yes. But this is very different. We just draw blood.

 I see.

 Can you take off your jacket?

 Sure. Is it better to take off my shirt, too?

 The sleeve of your shirt is not tight so it is OK.

 I see. Which arm do you prefer?

 Let me see … We can see your veins well for giving blood. Either arm will do.

 Then, please use my left arm.

 All right. Let me wrap your arm with this rubber band.

 Yeah.

Are you allergic to rubbing alcohol?

 No, I don't think so. They always rub my arm with sterile cotton before giving injections.

 I see. Let me rub your arm. Please make a fist with your thumb in.

 Okay.

 It may sting a little.

 Okay.

 You don't have any numbness in your fingers?

 No.

 Now we are finished. Please press this gauze here for a while. The results will be ready by next Tuesday.

 It will be ready by when?

 Next Tuesday, when you have an appointment to see the doctor.

 Oh, yes, yes.

 He will explain the results of the blood test at that time.

 I see. Thank you.

 I hope you get well soon.

Additional Medical Expressions

31 Are you allergic to rubbing alcohol?
消毒用アルコールにアレルギーはありますか？

32 You don't have numbness in your fingers?
指はしびれていませんね？
Don't you have…？ だと押しつけがましいので平叙文で尋ねています。

33 Please press this gauze here for a while.
しばらくこのガーゼを抑えておいてください。

34 The results will be ready by next Tuesday.
結果は次の火曜までに出ます。
ready で結果を知らせる準備ができることをいいます。

Let's Use Communication Strategies！

相手の言ったことの一部を聞き直す CS

　相手の言ったことの一部が聞き取れないときにどの部分がわからなかったか明確にして聞き返す CS です。

例1）p.46-l.4

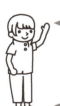

Does anyone have the number card two-one-four?

The number two-one-what?

Two-one-four.

番号の一部が聞き取れなかったので，その部分を what にして「2-1-何番？」

と聞いています。

例2) p.46-l.17

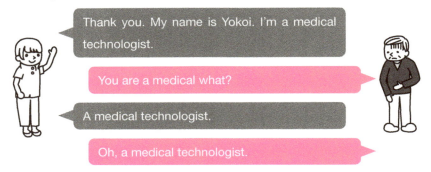

自己紹介で言われた職種の一部，a medical の後が聞き取れず，technologist の部分を what にして聞き返しています。

例3) p.48-l.13

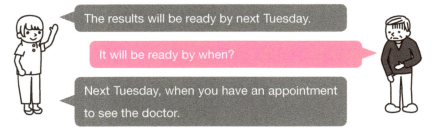

いつまでに結果が出るか言われたが，肝心の曜日が聞き取れなかったため，曜日の部分に when を入れて「いつまでに出るって言ったの？」と聞き直しています。

B Medical Reading

Medical Terminology

anemia	貧血	living tissue	生体
antigen	抗原	magnetic resonance imaging (MRI)	磁気共鳴映像法
bacteria	細菌	malignant	悪性の
compatibility	適合性	medical radiation technologist (MRT)	診療放射線技師
cultivate	培養する		
digestive	消化器の	microbe	微生物
electrocardiogram (ECG)	心電図	physiological	生理学的な
electroencephalogram (EEG)	脳波図, 脳電図	protein	タンパク質
		pulmonary function test	呼吸機能検査
electromyogram (EMG)	筋電図	red blood cell	赤血球
funduscopy	眼底検査	specimen	検体
gene	遺伝子	transplant	移植
germ	病原菌	ultrasound	超音波
hormone	ホルモン	vitamin	ビタミン
invasive	侵入する, 侵略的な	white blood cell	白血球

Medical Technologist (臨床検査技師)

　The duty of a medical technologist (MT) is analyzing patients' specimens including living tissues with other information to report the finding to doctors and dentists. An MT's job is carried out following the doctors or dentists' directions.

　An MT's analysis of the various specimens is mainly performed in a laboratory. General examination of urine and feces can reveal abnormality of the kidney, liver or other digestive organs. Blood tests may suggest various conditions such as anemia or inflammation by the quantity or quality of red blood cells or white blood cells, or abnormalities of our organs by measuring levels of sugar, proteins, vitamins, hormones, drugs etc. MTs can find invasive germs such as bacteria or viruses in the blood by examining the presence of antigens and antibodies. Moreover, they often cultivate samples of urine, feces, blood or phlegm to detect the existence of some microbes. Examinations of the tissues from our organs may show the existence of malignant cancer cells. It is also MTs' responsibility to examine a patient's DNA to detect abnormalities in the genes, to match blood for transfusions or to check compatibilities of transplants.

Besides specimen tests in a laboratory, MTs are responsible for conducting physiological function tests: for example, an electrocardiogram (ECG), electroencephalogram (EEG), pulmonary function test, electromyogram (EMG), funduscopy, ultrasound, magnetic resonance imaging (MRI) and others, although in some institutions, medical radiation technologists (MRTs) may perform an ultrasound or MRI. MTs need to read and evaluate these images precisely to correctly assist in the doctors' diagnosis or treatment of a patient. Therefore they are required to have at least three years of college or vocational school and pass the national test. Even after they are licensed, they need to continue to update their studies to be true professionals in their field.

Comprehension

1) 本文の内容について，次の問いに英語で答えなさい。
1. Where do MTs primarily work to analyze specimens?
2. What elements of blood are examined to diagnose anemia or

inflammation?
3. Why do MTs cultivate samples?
4. What is examined to show the existence of malignant cancer cells?
5. What physiological function tests are performed by MTs?
6. How many years does one have to study at school to be an MT?

2）本文の内容に合うように語群より適切な語句を選び，（　　）内に入れなさい。

(1) and feces are effective specimens to understand the abnormality of the kidneys, liver or other (2) organs. Abnormalities of our organs can be detected by measuring levels of sugar, (3), vitamins, hormones, drugs etc. or invasive germs such as (4) or viruses shown by the presence of (5) and antibodies in the blood sample. MTs also examine the patient's DNA to detect abnormalities in the (6), to match blood types for (7) or to check compatibilities for (8).

| antigens | bacteria | digestive | genes |
| proteins | transfusions | transplants | urine |

ほっと一息！

　　electrocardiogram（ECG），electroencephalogram（EEG），electromyogram（EMG）など -gram が histogram（柱状グラフ），hologram（ホログラム），phonogram（表音文字）などと同様，図の意味だということはわかりましたね。他に，重さの単位の「グラム」やグラム陰性，グラム陽性などという細胞の染色法の「グラム」もありますが，別の語源だと考えられます。

Helpful English Grammar

1. of の用法：〜 of … = …の〜

analysis **of** the various specimens	種々の検体の分析
general examination **of** urine and feces	尿や便の一般的な検査
abnormalities **of** our organs	器官の異常
the existence **of** some microbes	ある微生物の存在
compatibilities **of** transplants	移植の適合性

of を含む意味の塊（句）は多くの場合，of の後と前を「〜の」でつなげば適切に解釈できます。ただし，another kind of examination「別の種類の検査」のような用例もあるので **of を含む慣用句は例外**として覚えていきましょう。of の前後でひとかたまりの表現（句）としてとらえると，文の構造を考えるときの助けにもなります。

2. 副詞の用法：副詞は動詞，形容詞，副詞，文全体を修飾します。今回は動詞を修飾する例で考えましょう。

MTs' analysis of the various specimens **is mainly performed** in a laboratory.

　臨床検査技師の種々の検体の分析は検査室で**主に行われている**。

It **is also** MTs' responsibility to examine the patient's DNA.

　患者の DNA を検査すること**もまた**，臨床検査技師の責務**である**。

MTs need to **read and evaluate** these images **precisely** to **correctly assist** in the doctors' diagnosis or treatment of a patient.

　医師の患者の診断や治療を**正しく補助する**ために臨床検査技師は**正確に**これらの画像を**読み，評価する**必要がある。

ほっと一息!

　血液検査結果の数値の単位に注目したことがありますか。一般的な血液検査で目にする赤血球、白血球、血小板などに関わる検査項目と生活習慣病に関係のある項目から脂質、糖質の数値とその単位を確認してみましょう。

血液検査項目	略号	基準範囲	単位
赤血球数	RBC	男性　400-539 女性　360-489	$10^4/\mu L$
白血球数	WBC	3.2-8.5	$10^3/\mu L$
血小板数	PLT	13.0-34.9	$10^4/\mu L$
血色素量	Hb	男性　13.1-16.6 女性　12.1-14.6	g/dL
ヘマトクリット	Ht	男性　38.5-48.9 女性　35.5-43.9	%
HDL コレステロール（善玉）	HDL-C	40-119	mg/dL
LDL コレステロール（悪玉）	LDL-C	60-119	mg/dL
中性脂肪（トリグリセリド）	TG	30-149	mg/dL
空腹時血糖（fasting plasma glucose） ヘモグロビン・エーワンシー（NGSP）	FPG HbA1c	-99 かつ -5.5＊	mg/dL %

出典：日本人間ドック学会／人間ドック判定・指導ガイドライン作成委員会による「判定区分」表（2014年4月1日改訂, http://www.ningen-dock.jp/other/inspection）
＊99以下かつ5.5以下を表す。

　赤血球，白血球，血小板はそれぞれ「数」なので，何個あるかということになります。たとえば白血球は1マイクロリットル中に3.2×1000個〜8.5×1000個あれば基準範囲にあり，問題ありません。血色素，HDL コレステロール，LDL コレステロール，中性脂肪，空腹時血糖の基準範囲はそれぞれ1デシリットル中に何ミリグラム入っているかで判断されます。ちなみに英語ではmilligram(s) per deciliter と読みます。ヘマトクリットや HbA1c の基準範囲はそれぞれ％の割合で示します。

Chapter 6
Internal Medicine: Diabetes
内科：糖尿病

　糖尿病を疑われるときの症状，検査について会話で学びましょう。
　糖尿病はインスリン作用不足による慢性の高血糖状態を主徴とする代謝症候群です。糖尿病は主に１型，２型，妊娠糖尿病，その他の糖尿病があります。自覚症状がほとんどないため，健康診断で指摘されることが少なくありません。糖尿病治療の基本には食事療法，運動療法，インスリンを含む種々の薬物療法などがあります。

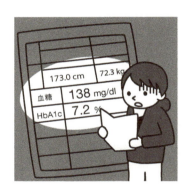

Purposes of this Chapter

臨床英語表現	糖尿病の症状・治療に関する表現
コミュニケーション・ストラテジー	相手の言った内容を自分が正しく理解しているかを確認する
医療従事者の知識	糖尿病についての正しい知識
重要構文	関係代名詞 that，前置詞＋関係代名詞，関係代名詞 which の継続用法，前置詞＋動名詞，neither A nor B

Medical Dialogue

Basic Medical Expressions

医療現場でよく使われる簡単な表現です。自然に言えるようになるまで声に出して何度も読み，完全に覚えましょう。

---

35 Why have you come here today?
今日はどうしたのですか？

---

36 It shows that I have suspected diabetes.
それには糖尿病の疑いがあると記されています。

---

37 Do any of your family members or relatives have diabetes?
家族や親せきに糖尿病の人はいますか？

---

38 Please come back in two days for the lab results.
2日後に検査結果を取りに来てください。

「検査」は medical test，「精密検査」は thorough examination と表現できます。in two days は「2日経ったら」で，in は after と同じ意味になります。

Medical Terminology

complication	合併症	nephropathy	ネフロパシー，腎臓症
fasting glucose level	空腹時血糖	OGTT（oral glucose tolerance test）	経口ブドウ糖負荷試験
frequent urination	頻尿	retinopathy	網膜症
HbA1c level	（グリコ）ヘモグロビン A1c レベル	suspected diabetes	糖尿病の疑い（糖尿病予備軍）
insulin secretion	インスリン分泌		
medical examination report	健康診断報告書		

Internal Medicine Department（内科）

　健（32 歳）の会社の同僚である山田（40 歳）が，先月健康診断を受け，昨日結果を受け取り，そこには糖尿病の疑いがあることが記されていました。健康に自信があった同僚はその内容に驚き，翌日，健康診断結果を持参して病院に来ています。内科受付で問診表に記入した後，診察を受けています。

▷ 医師は健の同僚にどのような質問をしているのでしょう。
▷ 健の同僚の健康診断の結果はどうでしたか？
▷ 医師は健の同僚にどんな忠告をしたのでしょう。

 Doctor: Why have you come here today?

 Yamada: Yesterday I received a medical examination report which I had a month ago. It shows that I have suspected diabetes but the other items of the medical examination are all good.

 Would you show me the medical examination report?

 Here you are.

 How has your weight changed recently?

 I have gained about 5 kg over the past couple of years. Perhaps it is because of taking more snacks and a lack of physical activities.

 Do you have any symptoms such as increased thirst, taking much water and frequent urination?

 No, I don't.

Your water drinking or urination hasn't changed recent years. Am I correct?

Yes.

 Do any of your family members or relatives have diabetes?

My mother and aunt do.

 Oh I see.

You mean I have hereditary diabetes?

 It is possible. Are you OK?

Yes. Both my mother and aunt look fine though they have diabetes.

According to your medical examination report, your fasting blood glucose level is 138 mg/dl, which is higher than normal. Your HbA1c level is 7.2% and also higher than normal. I need to run some blood tests in detail by means of OGTT (oral glucose tolerance test) of 75 g (a blood glucose level and the way of changing insulin secretion). More tests are needed to check whether you have some complications caused by diabetes, such as retinopathy or nephropathy. I will treat you considering the results of those tests.

You mean I have diabetes and need to be treated with medication?

No, you don't always need to be treated with medication. It depends on how the disease develops in the body. Diabetes is a chronic disease and keeping blood glucose level as normal or close to a normal situation is important. So it is necessary for people with diabetes to keep a normal body weight, exercise enough and take good nutrition. We have a class that a registered dietitian teaches to patients with diabetes about how to take a suitable diet for diabetes. You had better attend the class.

Additional Medical Expressions

(39) I have gained about 5 kg.
5キロくらい体重が増えた。
gain, put on は「体重が増える」。反対は lose weight です。weight scale は「体重計」。

(40) It is because of taking more snacks and a lack of physical activities.
間食の取りすぎと運動不足のためです。
because of は「〜のため」を意味し, of の後には名詞, 動名詞, 名詞句がきます。

(41) I will treat you considering the results of those tests.
検査結果を考慮して治療します。
considering 〜は分詞の慣用表現で,「〜を考慮して」を意味します。

Let's Use Communication Strategies！

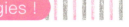

相手の言った内容を自分が正しく理解しているかを確認する CS

"Am I correct?" "You mean … ?" などの表現で自分の理解を確認できます。

Am I correct? 「それで正しいですか」の例:p.59-l.2

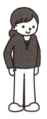
Your water drinking or urination hasn't changed recent years. Am I correct?(水分摂取と尿量に変化なしということで,正しいですか?)
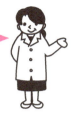

Yes.(はい。)

医師は自分の理解が間違っていないか,患者に確認しています。

You mean … ? 「つまり…ですか?」の例:p.59-l.8, 22

You mean I have hereditary diabetes?(つまり,私は遺伝性の糖尿病ということですか?)

It is possible.(可能性はあります。)

患者は医師の言ったことを自分の言葉で確認しています。

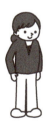
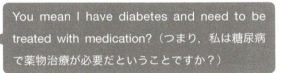
… I will treat you considering the results of those tests.(検査の結果から考えて治療します。)
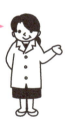

You mean I have diabetes and need to be treated with medication?(つまり,私は糖尿病で薬物治療が必要だということですか?)

ここでも患者は,医師が言ったことを確認しています。

このようなCSにより自分の解釈が間違っていないかを確認することは,医療従事者に特に求められます。

B Medical Reading

Medical Terminology

autoantibody	自己抗体	gestational diabetes mellitus	妊娠糖尿病
diabetes mellitus（もしくは単に diabetes と書く）	糖尿病	hemodialysis	透析
		hyperinsulinemia	高インスリン血症
diabetic nephropathy	糖尿病性腎症	insulin resistance	インスリン抵抗性
diabetic neuropathy	糖尿病性神経症		
diabetic retinopathy	糖尿病性網膜症	Langerhans island	ランゲルハンス島
		pancreas	膵臓

Type 2 Diabetes Mellitus（2型糖尿病）

Diabetes mellitus is caused by chronic high blood sugar level due to a shortage of insulin secretion or function. It is usually known as simple term "diabetes". Insulin is the only hormone that lowers blood sugar level and is secreted from β cells in Langerhans island of the pancreas and so the amount of insulin secretion is related to the diabetes' occurrence.

There are two causes of a deficiency of insulin. In spite of producing enough insulin, a kind of diabetes occurs, which is called "insulin resistance". In the case of a lack of insulin secretion, much more amount of insulin is sometimes secreted than that is necessary because the insulin effect is not good. The situation is called "hyperinsulinemia".

It is commonly known that obesity, stress and not enough body exercise cause insulin resistance.

Diabetes is divided into four types: type 1 diabetes mellitus, type

2 diabetes mellitus, gestational diabetes mellitus and other type of diabetes mellitus.

Type 1 diabetes mellitus occurs among infants and young people, the cause of which is absolute insulin deficiency owing to disruption of β cells caused by autoantibodies.

Type 2 diabetes mellitus is the body situation of a relative insulin shortage, which occurs among the middle aged people and is deeply related to obesity and life-style factors including high calories diet, lack of physical activity, stress and so on. Genetic factors are involved in the disease and the members in the same family and relatives often have type 2 diabetes mellitus.

Diabetes is diagnosed by the results of the examinations such as fasting plasma glucose level, 75 g oral glucose tolerance test, and HbA1c according to the diagnostic criteria made by the Japanese Diabetes Association.

The symptoms of diabetes are increased thirst, frequent urination, general fatigue, weight loss and unconsciousness in the case of extreme high blood sugar. In type 2 diabetes, symptoms are subtle for a prolonged period, so he or she doesn't notice the illness before receiving the result of a health examination.

Untreated diabetes leads to a variety of complications, in which the damage to a blood vessel is the major one. It is said that three major complications of diabetes are diabetic retinopathy, diabetic nephropathy and diabetic neuropathy. In Japan one in four over 40 has diabetes or suspected diabetes, 3000 people become blind every year due to the diabetic retinopathy and 15000 people start hemodialysis due to the diabetic nephropathy.

The basic treatments for diabetes are diet treatment, exercise treatment and medical treatment including insulin injection. Registered dietitians guide the patient how to get good nutrition for keeping a normal weight. It is necessary to take aerobic exercise for 15 or 30 minutes twice a day. When neither diet treatment nor exercise treatment shows sufficient effect for controlling blood glucose level, some medications will be considered.

Comprehension

1）本文の内容について，次の問いに英語で答えなさい。
1. What are some types of diabetes?
2. What are major causes of diabetes?
3. What do doctors diagnose diabetes by?
4. How is type 1 diabetes different from type 2 diabetes?
5. What are the good preventative measures for diabetes?

2）本文の内容に合うように語群より適切な語句を選び，（　）に入れなさい。

The symptoms of diabetes are as follows: (1), (2), frequent urination, whole body fatigue, and conscious disorder. Untreated diabetes leads to a variety of complications and the damage to (3) is the major one.

Three biggest complications of diabetes are (4), diabetic nephropathy and (5). The basic treatments for diabetes are (6), (7) and medical treatment including insulin injection.

diet treatment	increased thirst	a blood vessel
diabetic neuropathy	exercise treatment	weight loss
diabetic retinopathy		

Helpful English Grammar

1. 関係代名詞の that

　先行詞に **the only**, **all**, **最上級**, **序数**がついた場合，関係代名詞の **that** が好まれます。

Insulin is **the only** hormone **that** lowers blood sugar level.
　インスリンは血糖値を下げる**唯一の**ホルモンです。

Mary is **the kindest** woman that takes care of the elderly people.
　メアリーは高齢者の世話をする**最も優しい**女性です。

2. 前置詞＋関係代名詞：in which, of which, at which, for which

　前置詞の後には関係代名詞 **that** は**使用することができません**。

Untreated diabetes leads to a variety of complications, **in which** the damage to a blood vessel is the major one.
　糖尿病を治療しないといろいろな合併症を引き起こします。**合併症では**血管障害が大きなものです。

3. 〜 , which：関係代名詞の継続用法

　関係代名詞の継続用法では**前の文章全体**を示すことがあります。

Type 2 diabetes mellitus is the body situation of the relative insulin shortage, **which** occurs among the middle aged people.
　２型糖尿病は相対的インスリン不足の体の状態です。それは中年に発生します。

I didn't make preparations for English class, **which** made my teacher angry.
　私は英語の授業の予習をしなかった。そして**そのことが**先生を怒らせた。

4. 前置詞＋動名詞

　前置詞（in, on, at, for, of など）**の後ろの動詞は動名詞**（〜 ing）になり

ます。

In spite of producing enough insulin, a kind of diabetes occurs.

　十分なインスリン供給にもかかわらず，ある種の糖尿病が発生する。

He **is good at composing** music.

　彼は音楽を作曲するのが得意です。

Be careful **in crossing** the street.

　道を渡るときは気をつけなさい。

5. neither A nor B：AでもBでもない

When **neither** diet treatment **nor** exercise treatment effect for controlling blood glucose level, some medications are considered.

　食事療法でも運動療法でも血糖値制御に効果がないとき，薬物療法が考えられます。

I speak neither English nor Chinese.

　私は英語も中国語も話せない。

・上記と反対の表現

I speak **both English and Chinese**.

　私は英語も中国語も話せる。

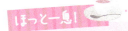

糖尿病の診断と患者数

糖尿病の臨床診断のためのフローチャートを図1に示します。

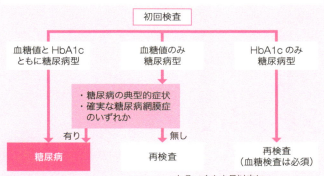

日本糖尿病学会糖尿病診断基準に関する調査検討委員会：糖尿病の分類と診断基準に関する委員会報告，糖尿病 55（7）：458，2012 より一部改変

図1 糖尿病の臨床診断のフローチャート

　世界の糖尿病患者人口は，アジア・太平洋地域において 2014 年から 2035 年では 1 億 3780 万人から 2 億 180 万人になると予測されています（表）。先進国ほど 2 型糖尿病が多く，2030 年台には患者が倍増すると考えられており，生活習慣，食の西洋化によりアジア，アフリカ，特に中国，インドにおける糖尿病人口が顕著に増加すると予測されています（図2）。

　日本では糖尿病が強く疑われている人は 2007 年にはおよそ 890 万人でしたが，2013 年には 950 万人に達しました（厚生労働省の国民健康・栄養調査より）。

表 世界の糖尿病人口予測（2014→2035年）

	2014年（億人）	2035年（億人）
アジア・太平洋地域	1.38	2.02
南アジア	0.75	1.23
北米	0.39	0.50
中南米	0.25	0.39
ヨーロッパ	0.52	0.69
アフリカ	0.22	0.42
中東・北アフリカ	0.37	0.68

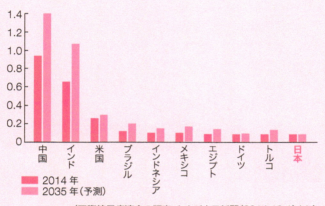

（国際糖尿病連合の調査，および中日新聞（2014.12.1）より）

図2 糖尿病人口の多い国

Chapter 7
Diabetes and Registered Dietitian

糖尿病と管理栄養士

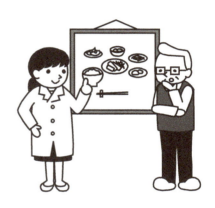

　糖尿病の食事治療のために管理栄養士から栄養指導を受けています。バランスの良い食事の取り方を会話で学びましょう。

　管理栄養士の仕事は病院での患者の食事指導，献立考案，学校での給食指導，地域における食事指導など多岐にわたっています。管理栄養士の役割を学びましょう。

Purposes of this Chapter

臨床英語表現	栄養療法に関する英語表現
コミュニケーション・ストラテジー	相手の理解を確認する
医療従事者の知識	管理栄養士と栄養指導についての正しい知識
重要構文	to 不定詞の目的，疑問詞＋to 不定詞，関係副詞の where

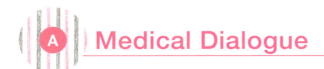

A Medical Dialogue

Basic Medical Expressions

医療現場でよく使われる簡単な表現です。自然に言えるようになるまで声に出して何度も読み，完全に覚えましょう。

---

42 You have only to take a well-balanced diet.
バランスの取れた食事をとればよい。

diet は栄養面からみた飲食物，治療のための規定食，減食の意味があります。「ダイエットをする」は go on a diet, be on a diet となります。

---

43 This may help you from eating too much.
食べ過ぎを防ぐ。

---

44 Eating moderately is the key to health.
腹八分目は健康の鍵です。

moderate は「適度な」，「節度のある」を意味します。反対に，過度な飲食は eat and drink too much, eat and drink excessively, excessive eating となります。

---

45 Type 2 diabetes is said to be related to a lifestyle-related disease.
2型糖尿病は生活習慣病と関係があるといわれています。

be related to ～：～と関係がある

Medical Terminology

business bachelor	単身赴任者	food substitution table	食物交換表
diabetic diet	糖尿食	grain	穀物
diet therapy	食事療法	ideal body weight	理想体重
feeling of fullness	満腹感	potential diabetes	糖尿病の可能性
food classification	食物分類	therapeutic exercise	運動療法

Nutritional Guidance for Diabetes（糖尿病の栄養指導）

　山田は先月受けた健康診断の結果を持って内科を受診しました。そこで2型糖尿病と診断され，医者から薬を飲む前に食事療法と運動療法をするように助言されました。今日はまず食事療法の指導を受けるため，病院内の栄養指導室に来ています（RD：Registered Dietitian）。

▷2型糖尿病を進行させないようにするにはどうすればいいのでしょう。
▷カロリー摂取量はどのように決められるのでしょう。
▷2型糖尿病患者は食事でどのようなことに注意すべきなのでしょう。

In a room for a nutritional guidance:

RD: Hello, Mr. Yamada. I will give you some guidance about a good diabetic diet.

Yamada: Thank you, I heard it from the nurse the other day. I will try to listen to what you tell me carefully.

RD: OK. You know there are different kinds of diabetes, for example type 1 diabetes and type 2 diabetes and others. Even when one has potential diabetes, he or she should take care of their body condition so as not to develop the disease.

Yamada: I was told I have type 2 diabetes.

RD: Type 2 diabetes is said to be related to a lifestyle-related disease due to deficiency of physical exercise, obesity, and environmental factor such as stress.

Middle-aged people are more likely to develop the disease than younger people. Diet therapy by being more careful about food and therapeutic exercise are important for the prevention of diabetes.

I will take a walk for one hour every day, but it is difficult to be careful about food because I am working away from my family in Tokyo, that is to say, a business bachelor.

 Don't worry, you have only to take a well-balanced diet, which is the most important.

That's difficult for me, isn't it? I wonder how much food I should take a day.

 Basically, the amount of energy needed a day is decided. The amount is calculated as follows: Ideal body weight (height(m) × height(m) × 22) × 25~30 kcal. For example, in the case of the person with a height of 155 cm, the ideal body weight is 52.8 kg. So the amount of energy needed a day is 53 × 25~30 = 1325~1590 kcal. This figure is the person's needed energy amount. You must take grain for 55~60% of the energy amount and food included protein for 25% of the energy.

Uuuuuh, it is very worrisome.

To put it shortly, eating moderately is the key to health. You can eat anything but the amount of food and the balance of the food is very important. You should take three meals a day regularly for the purpose of keeping your blood sugar level stable. Do you understand what I mean?

Yes, I do. Can I drink alcohol?

 No, you cannot. Alcohol and snacks are forbidden until you keep a good blood sugar level. Moreover you should eat anything slowly by chewing in order to get a feeling of fullness. This may help you from eating too much.

Oh, I see.

 We have a "food substitution table for diabetes therapy", which will help you take a good diet for diabetes. Food classification is written in this paper and please remember this.

I will try to take a good diet for my health. Thank you very much for your guidance.

 Please ask me whenever you have a trouble about diet for diabetes.

Food Classification

grain	protein	vitamin	mineral	dietary fiber
rice	meat	vegetables	dairy product	oatmeal
bread	fish	fruits	sea vegetables	natto (fermented soybeans)
noodles	egg			leaves of Japanese radish
potatoes	Tofu (bean curd)			burdock

Food Substitution Table

1 Unit＝80 kcal

Food classification	Food type	Distribution Examples of 20 Unit
Table 1	grains, potatoes, beans (except soybean)	11.0 unit
Table 2	fruits	1.0 unit
Table 3	fish, meat, egg, cheese, soybeans	4.0 unit
Table 4	milk, dairy food (except cheese)	1.5 unit
Table 5	oil and fats (include sesame, meat with much fat)	1.0 unit
Table 6	vegetables, seaweeds, mushrooms, konjaku	1.0 unit
Table 7	miso, sweet sake for seasoning, sugar	0.5 unit

Additional Medical Expressions

46 It is very worrisome.
不安です。
worrisome problem：やっかいな問題

47 That's difficult for me, isn't it?
それは私には難しいですね。
付加疑問の英文です。

(48)

I am working away from my family in Tokyo, that is to say, a business bachelor.

家族を東京において働いています。つまり，単身赴任なのです。

that is to say（つまり）で英文中に挿入される副詞節です。他に as it were（いわば），as far as … be concerned（…に関する限り）があります。

(49)

You should take three meals a day regularly for the purpose of keeping your blood sugar level stable.

血糖値を一定に保つために1日に規則正しく3食取るべきです。

「血糖値が上がる」は "The blood sugar level rises." "The blood level goes up." となります。

Let's Use Communication Strategies！

相手の理解を確認する CS

　自分の話している内容を相手が理解しているかどうか，時々確認しながら会話を進めることで，一方的な会話を回避できます。相手が会話を途中で遮ることを遠慮して，理解できないまま黙って聞いていることがあります。"Do you understand?" "Do you understand what I said?" "Do you understand what I mean?" などを使って本当に相手が理解しているのかを確認しながら会話を進めましょう。

血糖値を一定に保つために，一日3回規則正しい食事が必要だということを理解してくれたかな？

You should take three meals a day regularly for the purpose of keeping your blood sugar level stable. Do you understand what I mean?

Yes, I do.

　医療従事者は，時には非常に理解の難しい内容を説明しなければならないことがあります。そのようなときは，患者や患者の家族がこちらの言っていることを理解しているかどうか，確認しながら話を進めることが必要です。"Do you understand what I mean?（ご理解いただけましたか）"を日常会話でも使う練習をしましょう。

B Medical Reading

Medical Terminology

geriatric food	老人食	osteoporosis	骨粗しょう症
medical facility	医療施設（通例，複数形のfacilities）	potassium	カリウム
		the Ministry of Health, Labor and Welfare	厚生労働省
obesity	肥満	zinc	亜鉛

Registered Dietitian（管理栄養士）

　A registered dietitian（RD）is a license of the Ministry of Health, Labor and Welfare. RDs have two ways to get a license. One is that they work educating people about nutrition for a while after getting a dietitian license and have the national qualification examination of a registered dietitian. The other is that they study at university or training school which are admitted as an institution for training registered dietitians for three or four years. After graduating from the school, they can take the national qualified examination for a dietitian and a registered dietitian at the same time.

In Medical Facilities

RDs work in the medical facilities, elderly welfare facilities, community and educational facilities with the license of RD. The RD's profession requires high professional knowledge and food service management in order to take care of sick and wounded people and keep food safety standards and quality for meeting nutritional requirements.

RDs work in hospitals and health care facilities, where they offer diet therapy to many kinds of patients with physicians and other health care providers. They plan a hospital menu which is suitable for each disease, for example, diabetes, kidney disease, cardiovascular disease, obesity or osteoporosis, considering good food balance and the amount of energy, salt, fat, sugar, potassium, zinc and other nutrients. They also give patients and their family dietary consultations and teach how to take suitable food for improving their health.

RDs also work in elderly welfare facilities where they plan special menus which are suitable for every case of elderly people. They include swallowing disorder menu and liquid food menu.

In the Community

RDs offer knowledge about food for babies or elderly people in the community. Recently more elderly people stay at their homes, so more RDs must visit their homes for educating geriatric food to the family or home helpers.

At Educational Facilities

RDs do large-scale food planning at kindergarten, preschool, elementary school and junior high school, where they make menus which meet health and nutritional requirements for children. Especially, it is very important for them to ensure safety and keep quality.

Besides educational facilities, RDs are responsible for providing good menus and educating about the safety of kitchens at company cafeterias, restaurants and so on.

In an aging society, more and more specialized RDs will be needed to promote people's health and taking care of sick people not with medicine but with suitable food for each person.

Comprehension

1）本文の内容について，次の問いに英語で答えなさい。
1. What are the duties of a registered dietitian?
2. How does a registered dietitian get a license of RD?
3. Where does a registered dietitian work?
4. What kinds of diseases does a registered dietitian make a menu for at a hospital?
5. What does a registered dietitian do in the community?

2）本文の内容に合うように語群より適切な語句を選び，（　）に入れなさい。

　管理栄養士は（　1　）から認可された資格で，栄養士の資格を取得後に栄養指導をしばらく行った後，管理栄養士の資格試験を受けることができます。（　2　）大学または専門学校で教育を受けた人は，栄養士と管理栄養士の資格試験を同時に受けることができます。管理栄養士は（　3　）に対する療養のための必要な食事提供，食べ物の安全性の維持などのため，高度な（　4　）を取得しなければなりません。今日，管理栄養士は医療施設，教育施設，地域で不可欠な医療人です。特に高齢化が進む現代，（　5　）をする高齢者が増え，老人食についての訪問食事指導がますます必要になっています。

専門知識	調理師養成指定	厚生労働省	在宅療養
文部科学省	国	傷病者	器具の扱い方
入院	健康な人	都道府県	
管理栄養士養成指定			

Helpful English Grammar

1. 疑問詞＋to 不定詞

how to ～：どのように～すべきか（～の方法）

when to ～：いつ～すべきか

which to ～：どちらを～すべきか

what to ～：何を～すべきか

how to take suitable food

　適切な**食事の取り方**

His parents taught him **how to** study.

　彼の両親は勉強の仕方を彼に教えた。

I know **when to** do it.

　私はいつそれをすべきかわかっています。

2. 関係副詞：場所を示す where

RDs work in hospitals and medical facilities, **where** they offer diet therapy to many kinds of patients with physicians and other health care providers.

　管理栄養士は病院や医療施設で働きます。**そして，そこで**彼らはいろいろな患者さんに医師や他の医療従事者とともに食事療法を行います。

　関係代名詞でも表現できます（where ＝ in which, at which, on which）。

ほっと一息!

Q 最近「薬膳料理」「薬膳レストラン」などの「薬膳」をよく目にしますが「薬膳」って何？

A 薬膳は中医学（伝統中国医学）の理論に基づいています。中医学によると体の陰陽のバランスが崩れると病気になると考えられています。薬膳はこのバランスを整えるために，日々の食生活を通して行う飲食療法のことです。「薬食同源」という言葉がありますが，食材と生薬は同じ自然の中で育ち，得られるものであるため，本来，食べものと薬は区別していませんでした。長い歴史の中で，病気の治療薬と食材が区別されるようになりました。

　薬膳の基本は，食する人の体質に合わせ，旬の食材を取り入れ，体に不調があるときは，不調を取り除いたり，緩和する食材を加えることです。たとえば，便秘の時には便通をよくするイチジク，冷えには生姜，目の疲れにはクコ，元気がない時は山芋，えびがよく効きます。なつめ，クルミはアンチエイジングのためによいとされています。

とっておきの薬膳茶の紹介!!　ぜひお試しください
ジャスミン，ライチ，クコのブレンド茶

ジャスミン…独自の香りが滞った気の巡りを良くし，落ち込みやイライラを解消しリラックスさせてくれます。食欲不振や胃の不快感に有効で，目と頭の働きを助けます。
ライチ…楊貴妃が好んで食べた果実です。脾を補い，不足している血をつくり，血の循環を良くし，消化吸収を高め，肌や髪に張りとつやを与えます。また，いらだつ気分を鎮めます。
クコ…滋養強壮，視力を回復させ，老化を遅らせるのに有効です。肝や脾の働きを高め，血糖値や血圧を下げる働きもあります。
なつめ…「1日に3個食べれば年をとっても老けない」といわれています。

Chapter 8
Orthopedics: Traumatic Fracture

整形外科：外傷性骨折

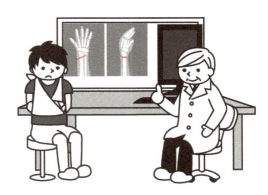

　転倒して痛みがある患者が受診した時の整形外科医と患者の会話例から，上肢の受傷の状況，受診時の疼痛の確認に使える英語表現，骨折の状況や治療方針，予後などを伝える英語表現を学びましょう。原因や状態による骨折の分類を確認するとともに，治療の一般的な考え方やリハビリテーションの必要性について基礎的な内容を英語で学びます。

Purposes of this Chapter

臨床英語表現	骨折の症状や治療に関連する表現
コミュニケーション・ストラテジー	相手の発言に簡単に感想を述べる
医療従事者の知識	骨折の主な分類や治療の基本
重要構文	分類を示す場合の be classified into/as，比較級の復習

A Medical Dialogue

Basic Medical Expressions

医療現場でよく使われる簡単な表現です。自然に言えるようになるまで声に出して何度も読み，完全に覚えましょう。

---

50 What is your problem?
どうなさったのですか？

受診理由を尋ねる目的で頻用される表現です。

---

51 Is it painful?
痛いですか？

臨床の必須表現です。Does it hurt? とほぼ同じ意味です。

---

52 Let's take X-rays and see.
X線写真を撮って見てみましょう。

Let's …（Let us の短縮形）で患者と医療従事者で一緒に何かをしようという感覚が表せます。

---

53 I will prescribe painkillers for three days.
痛み止めを3日分処方します。

「痛みの殺し屋（painkiller）」とは少々物騒ですが，わかりやすいですね。ちなみに除草剤は weed-killer といいます。

Medical Terminology

anesthesia	麻酔		fracture	骨折，折る
cast	ギプス		manipulate	処置する
CRPS（complex regional pain syndrome）	複合性局所疼痛症候群		orthopedics	整形外科
			painful	痛い
distal	遠位		painkiller	鎮痛剤
elbow	肘		proximal	近位の

radius	橈骨	severe pain	激しい痛み
rehabilitation	リハビリテーション，機能回復訓練	snap	ポキッという音
		wrist	手首
reset	整復する	X-ray	Ｘ線

Orthopedics（整形外科）

　三浦誠也（21歳）は，自転車で通学途中に道路で転倒しました。右腕を打撲して痛みが強いため，近くの病院で整形外科医の診察を受けています。

▷ どのような状況で転倒したのでしょうか。
▷ どの部分にどのような症状があるのでしょうか。
▷ 診断と治療について医師からどのような説明がなされたでしょうか。
▷ 誠也のその後の経過はどのように説明されたでしょうか。

Doctor: What is your problem?

Seiya: On my way to college, I was avoiding a passerby and fell off my bike. I landed on my right hand and I heard a snap in my wrist. I have had severe pain in my wrist since then.

Doctor: That's serious. Let me see. The wrist and the fingers of your right hand move normally but your wrist is swollen. Is it painful?

The doctor presses at the part 2-3cm proximal to the wrist, the distal end of his radius:

Ouch! Yes!

Oh, I'm sorry. ⋯ Your elbow and shoulder are normal. You may have a broken wrist. Let's take X-rays and see.

Seiya was led to the X-ray room and had X-rays taken of his right wrist:

According to the X-rays, you have a fractured radius in your arm.

That's terrible.

It is a simple fracture. The bones knit well especially in young people. An important thing is to reset the bone in the correct position.

Sounds painful.

Don't worry. We will use anesthesia when we manipulate it in place.

That's a relief.

Yes. If the bones cannot be reset well, we will need surgery to fix them with metal plates or pins.

I would feel as if I were a robot!

If we can reset the bones in the natural position, it would be kept in a cast so that it doesn't move.

 How long would I wear the cast?

 It takes about 4 to 6 weeks for the bone to knit together.

Seiya's bone was reset with anesthesia successfully and did not need invasive surgery:

 The bone is set to its normal position.

 That's great.

 You need to keep your arm in a cast for 4 weeks. After removing the cast, you will need some rehabilitation to prevent CRPS.

 What is that?

 Complex regional pain syndrome. That is when the fingers and wrist are swollen and you would have restricted or painful movement.

 I see.

 I will prescribe painkillers for 3 days. You can take them when you have severe pain.

 Thank you, Doctor.

Additional Medical Expressions

54 Your wrist is swollen.
手首が腫れています。
受動態を使います（swell-swelled-swollen）。

55 You may have a broken wrist.
手首が折れているかもしれません。
「折れた手首をもっている」と have で表現できます。

56 You need to keep your arm in a cast for 4 weeks.
腕を4週間ギプス固定する必要があります。
「cast の中に保つ」でギプス固定することをいいます。

Let's Use Communication Strategies !

簡単な感想，意見を述べる CS

That's serious.（p.83-l.13） ／ That's terrible.（p.84-l.10） ／ Sounds painful.（p.84-l.14）／ That's a relief.（p.84-l.17）／ That's a long time. ／ That's great.（p.85-l.9）

　That's や Sounds に形容詞，または名詞・名詞句をつけて相手の発言に共感を示したり感想を述べたりすると，その反応に応じた会話が発展します。

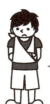

According to the X-rays, you have a fractured radius in your arm.

That's terrible.

It is a simple fracture.

　医師は橈骨骨折を告げられた患者の反応を見て，単純骨折であり，年齢的に

も治癒しやすい…という幾分楽観的な情報を最初に提供しています。しかし，たとえば，もし患者がここで "That's nothing." などと答えたら，医師は単純骨折だけど整復が上手くいかない場合のことを強調するなど，患者の楽観視を牽制することになるのではないでしょうか？

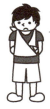
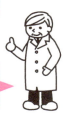

> An important thing is to reset the bone in the correct position.

> Sounds painful.

> Don't worry. We will use anesthesia when we manipulate it in place.

> That's a relief.

ここでは医師が骨折部位の整復をすることを述べたのについて，患者から痛そうだという感想が述べられたため，医師は麻酔を使用することを説明しています。それを聞いて患者が安心したのを確認して，医師は話を進めていきます。

簡単な CS ですが，相手の言うことへの関心を示すことにより会話を発展させるのに威力を発揮します。医療従事者としても利用価値は高いはずです。

Medical Reading

Medical Terminology

affect	侵す	continuity	連続性
bone tumor	骨腫瘍	contracture	拘縮

crack	ひび，亀裂	stress fracture	疲労骨折
immobilize	固定する	tolerance	耐性
impose	課す，負わせる	traumatic fracture	外傷性骨折
pathological fracture	病的骨折		

Fracture（骨折）

Fractures are classified into three types by the cause: traumatic fracture, pathological fracture and stress fracture. A fracture caused by force which is stronger than the tolerance of the normal bone is called traumatic fracture. For example, the fracture brought by falling down from a high position or being hit by a car is usually a traumatic fracture. Pathological fracture is caused when the bone is affected by diseases and fractures occur with slight force to the bones or joints. Osteoporosis is a well-known disease for this type of fracture and bone tumors are often found at near the fracture site. Stress fractures occur when stresses are repeatedly imposed on certain areas. Athletes usually train by repeating the same motion, which can be the location of a stress fracture. This sometimes troubles athletes because they must stop their usual training for weeks to cure the fracture.

Fractures are also classified as complete or incomplete fractures. In a complete fracture, the bone breaks into separate pieces whereas in an incomplete fracture, the bone retains partial continuity like a crack. The displaced complete fracture causing a wound under the skin is classified as a closed（simple）fracture. When fractures cause an open wound, they are classified as an open（compound）fracture. Open（compound）fractures have higher risks of infection and their prognoses can be worse than those of closed（simple）fractures.

Standard treatment is to reset the bones to their natural positions and immobilize them in a cast for about four weeks. Afterward, rehabilitation is necessary to prevent contracture of the joints or CRPS (complex regional pain syndrome) caused by the immobilization of the cast.

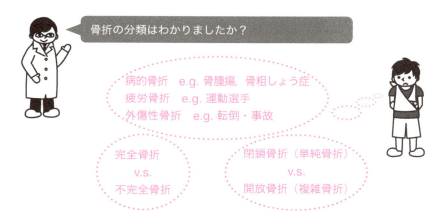

Comprehension

1）本文の内容について，次の問いに英語で答えなさい。

1. What fracture might often occur in elderly people due to loss of bone density?
2. What is the cause of stress fractures?
3. What is the fracture classification if the bone is not broken into separate parts?
4. What do you call the fracture if the broken bone breaks through the skin?
5. What fracture is most at risk for infection?
6. What procedures are typical in the treatment of closed fractures?
7. What is the purpose of rehabilitation in the treatment of a fracture?

2）本文の内容に合うように語群より適切な語句を選び，（　）に入れなさい。

　There are various major classifications of fractures. ① The cause is whether it is traumatic, (　1　) or stress to the bone; ② the type of fracture is complete or incomplete; and ③ if the fractured bone is under the skin called (　2　) or open (　3　).

　To treat the fractures, first, we (　4　) the bone to the original position, second, apply a (　5　) to keep the bone immobilized and third, have (　6　) to prevent contracture.

cast	compound fracture	pathologic	reset
rehabilitation	simple fracture		

Helpful English Grammar

1. be classified into …/ be classified as … : …に分類される

　解剖生理学，病理学等では分類に関する表記がよく見られます。分類の典型的な表現として "classify（分類する）" とその受身形の "be classified（分類される）" の表現に慣れましょう。

Fractures are classified into three types by the cause: traumatic fracture, pathological fracture and stress fracture.
　骨折は原因により3つの型に分類されている：外傷性骨折，病的骨折，そして疲労骨折である。

Fractures are also classified as complete or incomplete fractures.
　骨折はまた，完全あるいは不完全骨折に分類される。

2. 比較級の復習　「〜より…だ」「より…な〜」

　比較級は比較する対象を than の後ろに示す場合と省略される場合があります。一般的には strong-stronger, high-higher のように形容詞，副詞の語尾

に "er" をつけて比較級をつくりますが、例外的に bad-worse, good-better, little-less のように不規則なものもあるので覚えておきましょう。また、形容詞の場合、形容詞の原級の用法と同様に下記①のように名詞を修飾する場合（限定用法）と②のように補語として使われる場合（叙述用法）があります。

① Open (compound) fractures have **higher** risks of infection …

複雑骨折は**より高い**感染リスクを伴う。

② … their prognoses can be **worse** than those of closed (simple) fractures.

それらの予後は単純骨折の予後**より悪い**。

A fracture caused by force which is **stronger** than tolerance of normal bone is called traumatic fracture.

通常の骨の耐性**より強い**力で引き起こされた骨折は外傷性骨折と呼ばれる。

ほっと一息！

骨折の原因としては事故が多くを占めます。下図は厚生労働省によって3年に1回行われる患者調査を基に、骨折による入院・外来患者の割合をグラフにしたものです。骨折の原因（a）～（f）のうち、一番多い（c）は、「自傷」「他傷」「交通事故」「スポーツ中の事故」「転倒・転落」「その他の不慮の事故」のうちの何でしょうか。答えは下部にありますが、見ないで考えてみましょう。

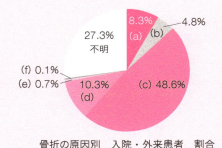

骨折の原因別　入院・外来患者　割合
出典：厚生労働省統計 平成23年患者調査

答え　(a) 交通事故　(b) スポーツ中の事故　(c) 転倒・転落　(d) その他の不慮の事故
　　　(e) 自傷　　　(f) 他傷

Chapter 9
Rehabilitation: Physical Therapist

リハビリテーション:理学療法士

骨折でギプス固定をしていた患者の骨折が治癒した後には,リハビリテーションが必要です。手首の骨折後のリハビリテーションの際の患者と理学療法士の会話で,関節を曲げたり伸ばしたりすることに関する表現を学びましょう。また,理学療法士の役割,活躍の場や対象とする人々,理学療法の実施方法の基本,理学療法士の資格取得までに学ばなければならない内容を読み取りましょう。

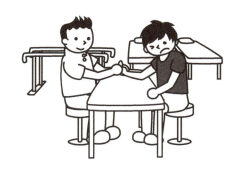

Purposes of this Chapter

臨床英語表現	リハビリテーションや理学療法士に関連する表現
コミュニケーション・ストラテジー	相手の発言をくり返す
医療従事者の知識	理学療法士の仕事
重要構文	分詞構文

Medical Dialogue

Basic Medical Expressions

医療現場でよく使われる簡単な表現です。自然に言えるようになるまで声に出して何度も読み，完全に覚えましょう。

---

57 Can you bend your wrist forward?
手首を曲げられますか？

手首を掌の方へ曲げるのを掌屈，手の甲の方へ反らすのを背屈と区別しますが，患者には掌屈を bend forward，背屈を bend back とわかりやすく伝えています。

---

58 Let's warm your wrist.
手首を温めましょう。

warm は形容詞の「暖かい」の他に動詞で「温める」の用法もあります。

---

59 Tell me if it hurts.
もし痛いようなら言ってください。

簡単ですが使いたい表現ですね。

Medical Terminology

bend	曲げる，屈曲する	stiff	堅い，硬直した
hot pack	温罨法，温パック	stretch	伸ばす，伸展する
mobility	可動性		

Rehabilitation（リハビリテーション）

右橈骨の単純骨折整復後，4週間ギプス固定をした誠也（21歳）のギプスが外れ，リハビリ室で PT（physical therapist）の指導によるリハビリテーションを始めます。

▶現在の状況を把握するためにどのような動きを観察しているでしょう。

≣▷痛みを伴うリハビリの前後にどのようなことがなされるでしょう。
≣▷自宅ではどのようにするとよいと言われたでしょう。

You have tried to move your fingers and elbow and shoulder of your right arm and there is no problem now.

Seiya

No, there are no problems. But my right wrist doesn't move at all.

Your right wrist doesn't move at all? Let me see… Okay. That is a normal condition.

That's normal…

Yes. You haven't used it for so long and it is stiff and difficult to move. That's why you need rehabilitation. Let's see how much mobility you have in your wrist now.

Okay, I'll try...

Try to bend your wrist back.

It really won't move.

Okay. You can only bend your wrist back a little. Can you bend your wrist forward?

I think so.

So you can bend it some… Next, can you move your hand from side to side?

I can move my hand from side to side a little bit.

 Very good. Now let's warm your wrist with this hot pack. Here you go.

 It feels warm and comfortable.

 Yes, it should feel nice. We'll try moving your wrist again after it warms up.

 OK.

After a while:

 Now, let's push your hand back. Tell me if it hurts.

 OK. ⋯ Ow! It's painful.

 I see, let's try bending it the other way.

 That hurts too! I think that's my limit.

 So, that's how it is, so far. So, now let's try moving your hand from side to side again.

 It really hurts! It's like my wrist is breaking again!

 Oh, sorry. Don't worry. That is to be expected — try a little more this way.

 That's enough!

Good. Why don't you try stretching it a little by yourself?

Stretching it myself? Wow, I can do it much better now than I could before your help.

There you are. But it will get stiff again later.

You mean I will have less mobility this evening than now?

Yes. So please try to exercise it yourself. Now was good timing, after you had warmed your wrist.

OK. I will exercise by myself later after I have warmed up my wrist.

Then please come again for rehabilitation the day after tomorrow.

The day after tomorrow. Okay.

See you.

Thank you very much.

Additional Medical Expressions

It feels warm and comfortable.

温かくて気持ちいいです。

I feel ～ でも OK ですが，ここでは少し客観的に伝えたい例と考えましょう．

61 Let's try bending it the other way.
もう一方に曲げてみましょう。

背屈と掌屈の 2 種類の屈曲をしているので，another ではなく，the other となります。

62 Why don't you try stretching it a little by yourself?
ご自分で少し動かしてみてください。

63 Let's move your hand from side to side again.
もう一度手を左右に動かしましょう。

from … to …は場所についても時についても使えます。今回は side「側方」から side「側方」へということなので左右にという意味です。

Let's Use Communication Strategies !

相手の言ったことをくり返す CS

まったく同じことをくり返す場合から表現を少し変えている場合まで，いろいろなくり返し方があります。

人称代名詞を変える以外はまったく同じ例：p.94-l.6

My right wrist doesn't move at all.

Your right wrist doesn't move at all?

表現は変えているが内容はほぼ同じ例：p.94-l.10, p.95-l.5

That is a normal condition.
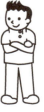

That's normal...

It feels warm and comfortable.

Yes, it should feel nice.

文の主要部分のくり返し例：p.96-l.3, 14

Why don't you try stretching it a little by yourself?

 Stretching it myself?

Then please come again for rehabilitation the day after tomorrow.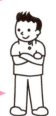

The day after tomorrow.

　新たな情報を提示するわけでないため、単純そうに見えますが、自分の理解に誤りがないか確認できるばかりか、表出された相手の思いに受容的、共感的態度を表すことができ、医療現場で不可欠な会話技法といえます。

 # Medical Reading

Medical Terminology

activities of daily living（ADL）	日常生活動作	electrotherapy	電気療法
adult day-care center	デイケアセンター*	immobility	動かないこと
		locomotive	運動の、移動の
anatomy	解剖学	locomotive syndrome	ロコモティブ症候群
assisted living facility	老人福祉施設*	nursing facility	介護（療養型）老人保健施設*
disabled	障がいのある		

＊「ほっと一息！」を参照。

passive movement	受動運動	relieve	軽減する
physiology	生理学	therapeutic	治療的な
quality of life (QOL)	生活の質	traction	牽引
		welfare facility	福祉施設

Physical Therapist（理学療法士）

　The primary purpose of the physical therapist（PT）is to relieve a patient's pain experienced when they move. They help patients to adapt or recover mobility to improve their activities of daily living（ADL）, which will in turn improve their quality of life（QOL）. Many PTs work with elderly people in hospitals, clinics, nursing facilities, assisted living facilities, adult day-care centers and clients' homes. Most patients need specific rehabilitation for difficulties in their daily activities though some do not have significant problems. Elderly people may have recreational training to prevent locomotive syndrome or complications which may lead to further immobility or injury, even if they have not suffered from serious diseases. Some PTs work for disabled children in welfare facilities, rehabilitation centers and/or in their homes, who need specific trainings to keep or promote their ADL. Other PTs work with healthy people or athletes, providing methodology for safe and effective training. Therefore, a PT's clients could be anyone from babies to elderly people, active healthy people or people in poor health. PTs need to adapt to distinct individual life styles and a variety of conditions.

　PTs help clients in their therapeutic exercise by manipulating passive movements of joints, muscle massage, traction therapy, electrotherapy, ultrasound therapy, warming or icing etc. To perform these therapies, a variety of knowledge and skills are required. They are required to pass a national exam after studying three or four years at specific training schools or colleges approved by the Ministry of Health, Labor and Welfare. They must learn the anatomy and physiology of the human body and diseases. They study internal medicine as well as orthopedic surgery to perform appropriate therapies. They also need to understand their clients' mental state to care for their clients properly. In utilizing a variety of physical therapies, PTs have to learn to do so much, but their hard work is worth it.

physical therapy は「身体の療法」？ それとも「物理的な療法」？

physical は mental の対義語としての「身体の，肉体の」という意味のほかに，「物理学の，理学の」という意味もありますね。physical therapy では物理的力や電気，温熱など物理的・理学的な方法を用いて治療することから「理学療法」といっていると考えてよいでしょう。

ちなみに occupational は「職業の」という意味が一般的ですが，occupational therapy では「職業」というより「作業」の方が実際の療法をよく表しており，作業療法と訳されています。

Comprehension

1）本文の内容について，次の問いに英語で答えなさい。

1. What are the main purposes for a physical therapist?
2. Where do most PTs work?
3. Who do PTs work with?
4. What kind of therapies do PTs perform with their clients?
5. How many years must they study before taking the national exam for PTs?
6. What knowledge and skills should a PT have?

2) **本文の内容に合うように語群より適切な語句を選び，(　　) に入れなさい。**

　　PTs work for (1) people either young or old. They also help people without any problems with their (2). PTs help their clients (3) their mobility or if they have pain, PTs try to (4) their pain. They utilize various therapies; passive (5) moving, muscle (6), traction therapy, electrotherapy, ultrasound therapy, warming or icing etc. For three or more years, they need to study about our (7) and bodies and a variety of physical therapies and pass the (8) exam to become a PT.

bone	boneless	disability	disabled	joint
joints	massage	massage	minder	minds
mobile	mobility	nation	nationality	relieve
relief				

Helpful English Grammar

分詞構文

　分詞構文は少しかたい表現なので会話ではあまり使われませんが，書き言葉では一般的に使われます。簡単にいえば，**接続詞**でつながれた文と同様な意味を，接続詞およびその後ろの**主語**を省略し，**動詞**を**現在分詞**（受動態では過去分詞または being ＋過去分詞）にして表す文です。たとえば，
The PT changed the rehabilitation plan, **when he saw** the patient's condition.

　この文の接続詞 when と主語 he を省略し動詞 saw を seeing とすると，同様の意味を表す次のような分詞構文になります。
The PT changed the rehabilitation plan, **seeing** the patient's condition.

　この分詞構文のみを見ると，省略された接続詞は because かもしれません

し，after かも，ひょっとしたら before あるいは as かもしれません。こうしたあいまいさは文脈からの判断に委ねられることになります。

　接続詞の意味を間違いなく伝えたいと思う場合は，**接続詞を残しておくこともできます**。たとえば，次の文では接続詞 after を残して，「3～4 年勉強後に国家試験受験」という時間的順序を明確に示しています。
They are required to pass a national exam **after studying** three or four years.

　接続詞 after と主語 they を補った文にすると次のようになります。
They are required to pass a national exam **after they study** three or four years.

Other PTs work with healthy people or athletes, **providing** methodology for safe and effective training.

　次の文は**接続詞と主語を補った**例です。
Other PTs work with healthy people or athletes **and they provide** methodology of safe and effective training.

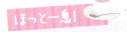

医療, 保健, 福祉の施設いろいろ

　Medical Reading の本文中に PT の活躍の場として hospitals, clinics, nursing facilities, assisted living facilities, adult day-care centers, clients' homes, welfare facilities, rehabilitation centers などの場所が出てきましたが, わかりにくかったと思います。これらを規定している法律を参考に整頓してみましょう。

hospitals：病院（医療法第1条の五：20人以上の患者を入院させるための施設を有するもの）

clinics：診療所（医療法第1条の五第2項：入院施設を有しない, または, 19人以下の入院施設を有するもの）。通称：クリニック, 医院等

nursing facilities：介護老人保健施設（介護保険法第8条27項：看護, 医学的管理の下で介護・機能訓練および生活の援助を行う）。治療が必要とされる保健施設を表すのに nursing を用いています。

assisted living facilities：介護老人福祉施設…治療ではなく生活援助が主であるため assisted living を使いますが, 自立や自宅での生活のための機能訓練もなされます。養護老人ホーム（老人福祉法第20条の4）や特別養護老人ホーム（介護保険法第8条26項）があります。

adult day-care centers：（高齢者向け）デイケアセンター, 海外で day-care というと, 幼児の保育をする施設を指すことが多いので気をつけましょう。介護保険法第8条8項で規定されている「通所リハビリ」の実施施設です。

clients' homes：介護保険法第8条5項の「訪問リハビリテーション」目的で PT が患者宅を訪問します。

welfare facilities：いわゆる特養（特別養護老人ホーム）も福祉施設ですが, Medical Reading では児童福祉法第42条に準拠した障害児入所施設を想定しています。

rehabilitation centers：Medical Reading ではリハビリ目的で通所する児童福祉法第6条2項3に基づく厚生労働大臣の指定医療機関を想定しています。

　こうした施設は各国の法律の規定や習慣により異なり, 日本独特のものもあることから, なるべくわが国の実情に沿う英語表現になるようにしました。

Chapter 10
Further Examination of the Lung: Lung Cancer

肺の精密検査：肺がん

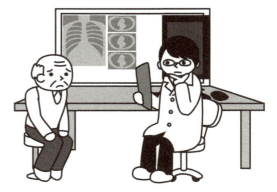

定期健診の結果から肺の再検査をすることになった患者と医師の会話から，問診内容，実施する検査とその結果，治療方法の説明に応用できる英語を学びましょう。また，原発性と転移性の肺がんについて概要を知り，原発性肺がんの代表的な組織型である扁平上皮がん，腺がん，小細胞がん，大細胞がんの特徴，肺がん発生の危険因子，治療法とともに早期発見の重要性についても読み取りましょう。

Purposes of this Chapter

臨床英語表現	肺がんの検査・治療に関連する表現
コミュニケーション・ストラテジー	理解を深めるために詳細を尋ねる
医療従事者の知識	原発性肺がんについての正しい知識
重要構文	関係代名詞の構文

Medical Dialogue

Basic Medical Expressions

医療現場でよく使われる簡単な表現です。自然に言えるようになるまで声に出して何度も読み，完全に覚えましょう。

---

64 Have you noticed any symptoms?
何かの症状にお気づきですか？
現在完了で尋ねています。

---

65 Do you smoke?
タバコは吸いますか？

---

66 How much did you smoke per day?
毎日どのくらいタバコを吸っていましたか？

Medical Terminology

adenocarcinoma	肺腺がん	lung field	肺野
anticancer drug	抗がん剤	lymph node	リンパ節
bronchoscope	気管支鏡	metastasis	転移
chemotherapy	化学療法	nodular shadow	結節性陰影
contrast CT	造影 CT	PET（positron-emission tomography）	陽電子放出断層撮影
CT（computed tomography）	CT 検査，コンピュータ断層撮影		
early-stage	早期の	PET-CT（または PET/CT）	ペット CT（PET と CT を同時に撮影する方法）
family history	家族歴（血縁者の病歴）		
		radiation treatment	放射線療法
general anesthesia	全身麻酔	recur	再発する
image	画像	right upper lobe	右上葉肺
incision	切開		

survival rate	生存率	well-differentiated lung cancer	高分化肺がん
video-assisted thoracoscopic surgery	胸腔鏡下手術		

Further Examinations for the Lung（肺の精密検査）

　三浦芳男（75歳）は定期健康診断で胸部異常陰影を指摘され，精密検査が必要となり，ある病院を受診しました。

▷芳男の喫煙歴はどうでしょう。

▷芳男の家族歴はどうでしょう。

▷芳男はどのような検査を受けたのでしょう。

▷この日のさまざまな検査の結果はどうだったでしょう。

In a consultation room:

 Doctor: What seems to be the problem?

 Yoshio: I need a thorough examination of my lungs due to the results of an annual medical examination.

 Doctor: Have you ever been told that you had something wrong with your lungs?

 Yoshio: No. This was my first time.

 Doctor: Have you noticed any symptoms?

 Yoshio: No, I have not noticed anything wrong. I've never had any diseases. I feel healthy.

I'd like to ask you about smoking. Do you smoke?

I started smoking when I was 20 and I quit when I was 65. After that I haven't smoked.

 How much did you smoke per day?

Well, about 20 cigarettes per day.

 I need to know a bit about your family history. Has anyone in your family had a serious disease?

I've heard my grandfather died of lung cancer. Other than that I haven't heard of anything.

 Okay. Let's begin.

What examinations should I have?

 First, we will do a blood test, then X-rays and CT scans.

Explanation of the blood test, X-rays and CT results:

 There's no problem according to the results of the blood test. The X-ray shows a small nodular shadow on the right upper lung field.

How was the CT scan?

According to the CT scan, a 15 mm pale shadow was found in the right upper lobe. This shadow could be cancer from the images but we need to perform bronchoscope, contrast CT and PET-CT for a definite diagnosis.

Explanation of the results after having CT and PET-CT:

 The results of the examinations show that you have adenocarcinoma.

Is it a cancer?

 Yes. It is in its early-stage and hasn't spread to lymph nodes but we need to start your treatment right away.

What kind of treatment should I have?

 Surgery is most preferable in your case though general treatments for adenocarcinoma are radiation treatment, chemotherapy with anticancer drugs and a surgical operation.

Operation … that sounds scary.

 In your case, video-assisted thoracoscopic surgery will be performed under general anesthesia to remove the upper lobe. This surgery requires only a few small incisions of about 2 cm.

Oh really? How long would I be in the hospital?

A 10-day hospitalization is normal after this operation. Chemotherapy is not usually given if the cancer is a well-differentiated lung cancer.

 What is well-differentiated lung cancer?

 It is a type of cancer which does not spread.

 That's good. How often does the cancer recur?

 A 5-year survival rate after the operation is higher than 80%.

 That's great.

 Please tell us if you choose to have the surgery after you discuss it with your family.

After the consultation above, Yoshio had the operation. There was no metastasis and his treatment proceeded as scheduled. He doesn't have any symptoms or recurrences and is enjoying an ordinary life.

Additional Medical Expressions

67 Has anyone in your family had a serious disease?
ご家族で重大な病気になられた方はいらっしゃいますか？
anyone in your family が主部です。臨床で serious といえば「重症，重篤な」の意味で頻用されます。

68 There's no problem according to the results of the blood test.
血液検査の結果では，何の問題もありません。
according to ～「～によれば」を確認しましょう。

69 Surgery is most preferable in your case.
あなたの場合，手術が最も望ましいでしょう。

preferable は prefer の形容詞です。

70 A 10-day hospitalization is normal after this operation.
この手術のあと 10 日間の入院が一般的です。

hospitalization: hospital（病院），hospitalize（入院させる）の派生語です。

ほっと一息！

「ローブ」って…（1）

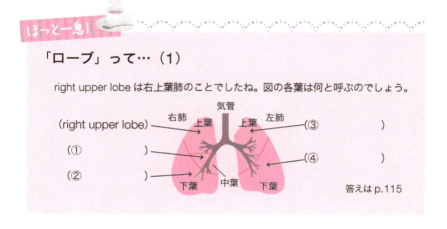

Let's Use Communication Strategies！

理解を深めるために追加の質問をする CS

相手に必要な情報を提供してもらう尋ね方として who, what, when, where, how などの疑問詞のある疑問文を使う例を見ましょう。

p.107-l.14

I started smoking when I was 20 and I quit when I was 65. After that I haven't smoked.

How much did you smoke per day?

喫煙について，さらに詳しい情報を聞き出そうとしています。

p.108-l.13

 we need to start your treatment right away.

What kind of treatment should I have?

ただちに治療を開始するという説明に対して，どのような治療か尋ねています。

p.108-l.21

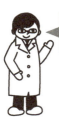 This surgery requires only a few small incisions of about 2 cm.

Oh really? How long would I be in the hospital?

軽微な手術だと告げられ，それなら入院期間がどのくらいか質問しています。

p.109-l.4

 ...if the cancer is a well-differentiated lung cancer.

What is well-differentiated lung cancer?

高分化肺がんの治療についての医師の説明に，それは何かを尋ねています。

p.109-l.6

It is a type of cancer which does not spread.

That's good. How often does the cancer recur?

転移しない型のがんだと聞いて，再発について質問しています。

相手の発言内容について疑問があればそのままにしないで尋ねることがコミュニケーションの基本です。疑問詞の疑問文はそのための便利な方法です。

 # Medical Reading

Medical Terminology

bronchi	気管支（bronchusの複数）	mutation	突然変異，変形
		pollutant	汚染物質
carcinoma	がん（上皮性の悪性腫瘍）	primary	原発性の
		proliferate	増殖する
epithelial	上皮の	small cell carcinoma	小細胞がん
large cell carcinoma	大細胞がん	squamous cell	扁平上皮細胞
metastatic	転移性の	trachea	気管
mucous membrane	粘膜		

Primary Lung Cancer（原発性肺がん）

　Lung cancers are classified into two types: primary and metastatic lung cancers. Primary lung cancer occurs in epithelial cells of the mucous membrane of trachea, bronchi and lungs. Metastatic lung cancer proliferates from malignant tumors which had entered blood stream from other organs. About 80% of lung cancers are primary lung cancers. The occurrence of lung cancers has increased year by year in both men and women and the rate of deaths by lung cancers is the highest of all cancers.

Primary lung cancers occur by mutations of genes of cells in lung tissues. The major tissue types of primary cancers are squamous cell carcinoma which is related to smoking, adenocarcinoma, which occurs most frequently in Japan, and small and large cell carcinomas, whose occurrences are less frequent.

Primary lung cancers, after early detection, are treated with a surgical operation. Regular medical examinations are important because few symptoms appear in early-stage lung cancers. Antismoking campaigns as in the US are said to have decreased the occurrence of lung cancers dramatically. An antismoking campaign in Japan may have similar results.

A relationship with smoking, air pollutants and occupational related dust has been proven to be risk factors for these diseases. Therefore, they can be prevented.

Comprehension

1) 本文の内容について，次の問いに英語で答えなさい。
1. What are two main types of lung cancers?
2. Where does primary lung cancer occur?
3. Which of the two types of lung cancers is most common?
4. What is important in treating primary lung cancer?
5. Which is the most related to smoking, carcinoma of a small cell, a large cell or a squamous cell carcinoma, or adenocarcinoma?
6. What cancer gives the highest death rate of all the cancers?
7. What are the risk factors for primary lung cancers?

2）本文の内容に合うように語群より適切な語句を選び，（　）に入れなさい。

　肺がんのおよそ8割は（　1　）で，気管・気管支・肺の粘膜上皮細胞の（　2　）の突然変異により発生するとされる。（　3　），大気汚染物質，職業的粉塵がこの（　4　）であることが証明されている。代表的な組織型には，喫煙と関係があるとされる（　5　）がん，最も発生頻度が高い（　6　）がん等がある。わが国の原発性肺がんは男女とも年々増加しており，早期発見，早期外科手術が原則であり，そのための定期検診が重要である。転移性肺がんは他の器官の悪性腫瘍が（　7　）で肺に運ばれ増殖するものである。

| 転移性 | 扁平上皮 | 血流 | 腺 |
| 原発性 | 危険因子 | 遺伝子 | 喫煙 |

Helpful English Grammar

関係代名詞

　ある名詞（先行詞）を説明するために that, which, who, whose, whom などの関係代名詞を使って説明する表現を続けます。関係代名詞は主語や目的語など文中での役割は異なってもその内容は先行詞と同じだと考えます。

例1）This is **the song which** I like very much.

　この文では **the song** の説明として **which** I like very much を続けています。

例2）He is **the teacher who** taught me English.

　the teacher の説明として **who** taught me English が付け加えられています。

例3）Metastatic lung cancer proliferates from **malignant tumors which** had entered blood stream from other organs.

　この文では，**malignant tumors** に **which** had entered blood stream from other organs という説明を加えています。「転移性の肺がんは悪性腫瘍から増殖する」という前半の「悪性腫瘍」が which の内容で，「その悪性腫瘍は他の器官から血流に入った」という説明を付け加えていることになります。

例4) The major tissue types of primary cancers are **squamous cell carcinoma which** is related to smoking, **adenocarcinoma, which** occurs most frequently in Japan, and **small and large cell carcinomas, whose** occurrences are less frequent.

　ちょっとややこしいですが，**a squamous cell carcinoma** に **which** is related to smoking という説明，**adenocarcinoma** に **which** occurs most frequently in Japan という説明，**small and large cell carcinomas** に **whose** occurrences are less frequent という説明がつけられています。

「ローブ」って…（2）

　p.110 の葉は① right middle lobe，② right lower lobe，③ left upper lobe，④ left lower lobe だとわかりましたね。lobe とはこうした葉（よう）のことで，肝臓に右葉（right lobe），左葉（left lobe），方形葉（quadrate lobe），尾状葉（caudate lobe）という名称があります。耳たぶのことを ear lobe ということから何となくイメージがわきませんか？

　日本語でローブというと lobe か robe かわからないので，間違えそうですね。ちなみに robe とは裁判官の法衣や欧米の大学の卒業式で着られるアカデミックドレスから bathrobe（バスローブ）や赤ん坊や女性の裾の長いゆったりしたワンピース式の服などの衣類をいいます。r と l を聞き分けるのが難しければ，まず発音の仕方から覚えておくといいですね。

r の発音の仕方：舌の先を上顎につかないようにして舌先を前から後ろに動かしながら息を出します。口は少しすぼめた感じです。
l の発音の仕方：舌の先を上の前歯の歯茎の後ろにつけて息が舌の左右から出るようにします。

　練習したら，英語の母語話者に聞いてもらいましょう。

Chapter 11
PET-CT Scan: Medical Radiation Technologist

PET-CT スキャン：診療放射線技師

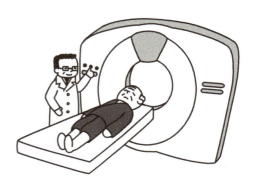

　診療放射線技師は，検査の種類によって検査前に注意事項の説明や必要事項の確認をする必要があります。PET-CT を受ける患者と診療放射線技師の会話でどのようなことを説明し，尋ねているかを学びましょう。診療放射線技師が提供する情報は医師の診断や治療に不可欠なものです。骨や関節，胸部，腹部の X 線写真でどのようなことがわかるのでしょう。また，CT，MRI の特徴や目的についても読み取りましょう。（注：診療放射線技師を示す英語としては，"medical radiological technologist" の方がより正しい）

Purposes of this Chapter

臨床英語表現	画像診断のうち PET-CT の実施に関連する表現
コミュニケーション・ストラテジー	理解を助けるために例示を求める
医療従事者の知識	診療放射線技師についての正しい知識
重要構文	another と other，such as の用例

Medical Dialogue

Basic Medical Expressions

医療現場でよく使われる簡単な表現です。自然に言えるようになるまで声に出して何度も読み，完全に覚えましょう。

---

71 Would you tell me your full name and date of birth, please?
お名前と生年月日を教えてくださいませんか？

Do you …? より丁寧な表現である Would you …, please? は患者に対してよく使われます。

---

72 Would you put on this gown?
この検査着を着てください。

「身に付ける」の意味で put on は広く使われます。

---

73 Would you take off your slippers and lie on this bed?
スリッパを脱いでこのベッドに寝てください。

take off は put on の対義語です。

Medical Terminology

dizzy	目まいがする，ふらふらする	radiology	放射線学
drowsy	眠い，物憂い	pollutant	汚染物質
		primary	原発性の
incorrectly	間違って，不適切に	proliferate	増殖する
muddled	混乱した	squamous cell	扁平上皮細胞
painless	痛みのない	trachea	気管

PET-CT Scan

　芳男（75歳）は胸部レントゲン写真やCT検査で異常が見つかり，悪性腫瘍が否定できなかったため，さらにPET-CT検査をすることになりました。検査に際し，診療放射線技師（MRT）がCT検査室で芳男に注意事項を説明しています。

▶ MRTは芳男に氏名や生年月日を尋ねる理由をどう説明していますか。
▶ 検査前の生活について，MRTはどのようなことを尋ねているでしょう。
▶ 検査前の準備としてどのようなことをMRTは伝えているのでしょう。
▶ 芳男の不安に対してMRTはどのように対応しているのでしょう。

MRT: Hello, Mr. Miura. I'm a medical radiation technologist. Would you tell me your full name and date of birth, please?

Yoshio: Good morning. I'm Yoshio Miura. I was born on June 21st, 1940.

Good.

Why do you always ask me my name and date of birth? You have that information, don't you?

Yes, we do. But we want to be sure not to make mistakes.

Mistakes? What kind of mistakes? Could you give me an example?

OK. Well, some people may be sleepy or drowsy when they take examinations. Other patients may have taken medicine before the examination which can make them muddled or dizzy. Perhaps people may answer incorrectly "yes" if they can't hear well or understand well. But if they are asked their name and date of birth, they usually answer correctly. Then we would not give the examination to the wrong patients.

I understand.

Good. Let me ask you some questions. Have you eaten anything this morning?

No. I was told not to eat anything after dinner on the previous day.

That's good. Did you have anything to drink?

I had several things to drink.

For example?

I drank water and had some tea.

Did you drink juice, soft drinks or milk?

No. Only water and green tea.

That's good. Have you had a flu vaccination in the past week?

No.

 Thank you. Now, I will explain the examination. You will wear a gown for the examination and a radiology doctor will ask you some questions. Then a nurse will give you an injection. You can drink water or green tea and you can go to the restroom but please quietly wait for an hour before the PET-CT.

I see.

Would you put on this gown and these slippers in the locker room? If you are wearing accessories, please take them off. When you are ready, please go to the next room to see the radiology doctor.

Can you give me an example? What can I wear under the gown?

Basically you cannot wear anything except your underpants.

Should I take off my watch or wedding ring?

Yes. That too. Just keep everything in the locker and be sure to lock the door. I'm in the next room so if you have any questions, please call me.

I think I understand. Thank you.

Yoshio is resting after seeing the doctor and having had an injection:

Hi, Mr. Miura. Are you feeling OK?

This is my first time to have a CT examination and I'm worried about it.

 I know how you feel. But PET-CT is painless and will be finished in about 20 minutes while you are lying on the bed. Do you need to go to the restroom? It will take about 20 minutes for the examination.

No. I have just been to the restroom.

 OK. Would you come this way, please?

Sure.

 Would you take off your slippers and lie on this bed?

All right.

 Would you put your arms over your head?

Like this?

 Yes. Very good. Please relax on the bed, though this is probably not as comfortable as your own bed.

It is a little cold but at least it is clean, right?

 That's true. Now we are going to start the PET-CT. Please do not move for about 20 minutes.

OK.

You can speak if you need to. I can hear your voice in the next room.

That's a relief.

 Please do not move until I say it's okay.

Additional Medical Expressions

74 Have you eaten anything this morning?
今朝，何か召し上がりましたか？
現在完了で尋ねています。

75 If you are wearing accessories, please take them off.
アクセサリーを付けていらっしゃるなら，外してください。
状態のようですが wear は進行形でも使います。

76 Do you need to go to the restroom?
トイレに行かなくてもよいですか？

Let's Use Communication Strategies!

理解を助けるために例示を求める CS

相手の発言内容がよくわからない場合でも，例を挙げてもらえばわかることがあります。そのような場合に例を挙げてくれるように頼む CS です。

p.118-l.20

 But we want to be sure not to make mistakes.

Mistakes? What kind of mistakes? Could you give me an example?

患者の氏名や生年月日などわかっているはずなのに，間違いを避けるために尋ねる臨床検査技師に対し，どのような間違いがあるのか例を挙げてもらっています。

p.119-l.17

I had several things to drink.

For example?

どのようなものを飲んだかを知るために，例を挙げてもらっています。このように具体的なことを尋ねた方が相手が答えやすいこともあります。

p.120-l.13

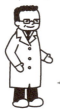 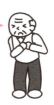

Can you give me an example? What can I wear under the gown?

Basically you cannot wear anything except your underpants.

検査着の下に何を身に付けていてよいか尋ねる文に続けて，例を挙げてもらおうとしています。

概念的なこと，包括的なことを答えて欲しい時もありますが，今回のCSを活用して具体例を挙げてもらうことで解決することもありそうですね。

B Medical Reading

Medical Terminology

angiography	血管造影	barium	バリウム

blood vessel	血管
bone scintigraphy	骨シンチグラフィ
cerebral	脳の
contrast enhanced CT	造影 CT
contrast medium	造影剤
digital imaging	デジタル画像
duodenum	十二指腸
electron beam	電子ビーム
esophagus	食道
exposure	（放射線）被曝
hemorrhage	出血
ileus	腸閉塞
intestine	腸

magnetic resonance	磁気共鳴
magnetism	磁気
MRI（magnetic resonance imaging）	磁気共鳴画像，断層撮影装置
nuclear medicine scan（または radioisotope examination）	核医学検査
ovary	卵巣
pulmonary	肺の
radiation	放射線
ulcer	潰瘍
ultrasonography	超音波検査（法）
urinary	泌尿器の
uterus	子宮

Medical Radiation Technologist（診療放射線技師）

The primary duty of medical radiation technologists（MRTs）is to provide and interpret digital image scans for a doctor's diagnosis and treatment. They are also responsible with the doctors, giving radiation treatments to patients with malignant tumors. MRTs utilize radiation such as X-rays and electron beam.

It is well-known that MRTs use X-rays to see fractures or other diseases of the bones or joints. Bone scintigraphy is another nuclear medicine scan which is especially useful to examine metastases. However, they are not the only targets of an MRT's job. They scan all organs and regions of the human body with a variety of devices. For example, they take X-rays of chest to detect tuberculosis, pneumonia, lung cancer, or other lung diseases or heart disorders. When young children swallow something accidentally, they also take X-rays to see where the foreign objects may be located. X-rays of the abdomen show us images of gas in the intestines caused by ileus, and with the help of barium, they can find ulcers and cancers in the esophagus, stomach, or duodenum.

CT or computed tomography is important for an MRT's job. CT can make sliced images of our body, which is useful to see conditions such as a cerebral hemorrhage or various disorders of digestive, pulmonary or urinary organs. CT is sometimes utilized with a contrast medium, which is called contrast enhanced CT scan, differentiating from simple CT scans, and gives us more information about the conditions of each organ. Angiography is a contrast enhanced CT with contrast medium in the blood vessels.

Medical radiation technologists also use magnetism or ultrasound. MRI or magnetic resonance imaging can also give us sliced images of specific soft tissues such as the brain, uterus, the ovary and muscles without radiation exposure. Ultrasonography is more easily and frequently used to examine the liver, uterus, heart, blood vessels, breast and many other organs because it does not need a very large device as with CT or MRI scans.

Thus, medical radiological technologists utilize various technologies to examine our bodies. It might be difficult or impossible for doctors to diagnose correctly and to treat serious diseases or injuries without MRTs' expertise. Their job is indispensable in the modern medical field.

Comprehension

1）本文の内容について，次の問いに英語で答えなさい。
1. What are the duties of medical radiation technologists?

2. What parts or organs of the body are targeted by X-rays?
3. For what purposes would an MRT take X-rays of the chest?
4. What can we find by an X-ray of the abdomen?
5. What scan shows us slices of images of a cerebral hemorrhage?
6. What are the two main CT types called?
7. Which type of CT is angiography?
8. What is an advantage of MRI compared with CT?
9. Why is ultrasonography utilized more often than CT or MRI?

2）本文の内容に合うように語群より適切な語句を選び，（　　）に入れなさい。

　診療放射線技師は（　1　）・治療のために画像を読影し，医療従事者に情報を提供し，がん治療にも関わる。X線は骨折や腫瘍ばかりでなく，人体のすべての部位を対象とし，胸部X線では結核，（　2　），心臓疾患，腹部X線では潰瘍，（　3　），また，子供の事故として多い（　4　）などの状態を見ることができる。（　5　）は骨への腫瘍の転移を調べるのに有用である。コンピュータ断層撮影（CT）は（　6　）CTおよび（　7　）CTに代表されるが，後者ではより多くの情報が得られ（　8　）もその一種である。さらに診療放射線技師は（　9　）のない磁気共鳴画像やより簡便な（　10　）を用いた検査も行う。現代医療には診療放射線技師の業務は不可欠である。

造影	肺炎	腸閉塞	超音波	血管造影	誤飲
被曝	単純	診断	骨シンチグラフィ		

Helpful English Grammar

1. other と another

　other は「他の，別の」という意味で，another は an other だと考えれば「一つの」other ということがわかると思います。

fractures or **other** diseases of the bones or joints
　骨折あるいは骨や関節の**他の**病気
the liver, uterus, heart, blood vessels, breast and many **other** organs
　肝臓，子宮，心臓，血管，乳房，多くの**その他の**器官
Bone scintigraphy is **another** nuclear medicine.
　骨シンチグラフィは**もう一つの**核医学です。
tuberculosis, pneumonia, lung cancer, or **other** lung diseases
　結核，肺炎，肺がん，あるいは**その他の**肺の疾患

2. such as
　例を挙げるときに使える表現です。
specific soft tissues **such as** the brain, uterus, the ovary and muscles
　脳，子宮，卵巣，筋肉**といった**特定の軟らかい組織
radiation **such as** X-rays and electron beam
　X線や電子線**のような**放射線を利用します。

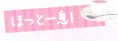

X線の利用

　X線の利用は医療分野のみではありません。たとえば，考古学的な価値のある物の内部を透視したり，絵画の下絵から真贋や作成過程を推測したりもできます。また，空港で預けた荷物や機内持ち込みの手荷物検査でもX線で透視しますね。乗客の検査でも金属探知機の他にX線を用いた全身スキャナーもあります。その他にもさまざまな場面で放射線が利用されています。

Chapter 12
Pediatrics: Bronchial Asthma

小児科：気管支喘息

　小児科医と気管支喘息が疑われる幼児の母親との会話から，症状や家族の病歴の尋ね方，治療方針，処方薬の説明の仕方を学びましょう。小児科の場合，家庭での様子については家族による観察が求められるため，その観察方法の指導も必要です。また，気管支喘息の発症の原因，経過，症状，検査，治療などについて読み取りましょう。

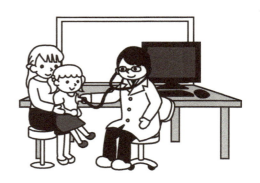

Purposes of this Chapter

臨床英語表現	小児科の代表的慢性疾患である気管支喘息に関連する表現
コミュニケーション・ストラテジー	相手に同意を求める
医療従事者の知識	気管支喘息とその薬物療法についての正しい知識
重要構文	過去分詞の形容詞的用法，受動態の用例

Medical Dialogue

Basic Medical Expressions

医療現場でよく使われる簡単な表現です。自然に言えるようになるまで声に出して何度も読み，完全に覚えましょう。

---

(77) How long has she been coughing?
彼女はどのくらい咳が続いていますか？
症状の継続期間なので，現在完了進行形を用いています。

---

(78) I cannot hear any abnormal sounds right now.
今は，異常な音はまったく聞こえません。
right now は now だけより時間を短く限定します。

---

(79) The results of the blood examination will be ready in about a week.
血液検査の結果は1週間くらいで出ます。
結果が出ることを「準備できる」としています。

Medical Terminology

allergy	アレルギー	pediatric	小児科（学）の
atopic	アトピー性の	pediatrics	小児科学
bronchial	気管支の	pollen	花粉
bronchodilator	気管支拡張薬	predisposition	（特異）体質，素因
dermatitis	皮膚炎	stethoscope	聴診器
inherited	遺伝の，遺伝形質の	wheezing	ゼーゼーいう音

Pediatrics（小児科）

加藤家のメイ（3歳）の長引く咳を心配した母親の洋子（30歳）が小児科を

受診しています。

▶ メイの咳について小児科医はどのようなことを洋子に尋ねていますか。
▶ 医師はメイの両親について何を，なぜ尋ねているのでしょう。
▶ 医師はメイが咳をしている時にどうするように洋子に言っているでしょう。
▶ メイの血液検査の目的は何でしょう。
▶ メイはどのような薬を処方されるのでしょうか。

In the pediatric consultation room in a hospital:

My daughter often coughs at night. We consulted a doctor at a clinic near my house. They said she has a cold and she took medicine but she isn't getting better. Could it be some serious disease?

 How long has she been coughing?

Almost two months. That is unusual, don't you think so?

 I think so too. That's highly unusual. She doesn't cough during the day, does she?

No. She rarely coughs in the daytime.

 Does she cough every night?

Not every night but at least three times per week.

 Does she cough when she falls asleep or early morning?

Well, she usually coughs just before morning.

Do you hear a wheezing sound when she is coughing?

Yes, I think I have heard something like that.

 She might have bronchial asthma from your description. Do you or her father have any allergies?

I have atopic dermatitis and my husband has a pollen allergy but no one in our families has asthma. I don't think she has inherited asthma. Do you think so?

 Yes, it's possible. Children often have bronchial asthma when their parents have experienced allergic reactions.

Really?

 Yes. I will have a look at her now.

After the examination:

 I cannot hear any abnormal sounds right now. Please listen to her breathing when she coughs at night.

But we don't have a stethoscope.

 You can hear it without a stethoscope.

I see. What should we be listening for?

 When she is coughing, put your ear to your daughter's chest or back. You will be able to hear a wheezing sound. So please try that when she is coughing.

I see.

 We may find out her allergic predispositions by means of a blood test. Do you mind if we draw her blood?

Of course not.

 I will prescribe a bronchodilator which is a medicine to expand her bronchi for a week. Let us know if the medicine helps her coughing get better. The results of blood examination will be ready in about a week.

I see. Thank you, Doctor.

Additional Medical Expressions

80
She doesn't cough during the day, does she?
彼女は昼間，咳をしないのですね？

81
Do her parents have any allergies?
彼女の両親にはアレルギーがありますか？
allergy（名詞（ǽlərdʒi））の発音に気をつけましょう。

82
Put your ear to your daughter's chest or back.
あなたの耳を娘さんの胸か背中に当ててみてください。
胸全体を表す chest を使っています。breast は主に胸の筋肉や乳房を，thorax は胸郭や胸腔を表します。

Let's Use Communication Strategies！

同意を求める CS

意見を求められると答えにくい場合も，同意するかどうかならば答えやすい

ものです。自分の考えに対する相手の意見を確認するための CS です。

p.130-l.13

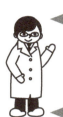

How long has she been coughing?

Almost two months. That is unusual, don't you think so?

I think so too. That's highly unusual.

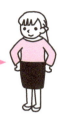

　小児科医の咳についての問いに，母親は 2 か月も続いているという事実とそれについての普通ではないと思う気持ちを述べています。そして医師にも変だと思わないかを Don't you think so?　と意見を求めています。今回は医師も普通ではないと思っていることを述べ，咳について話を深めていっています。

p.131-l.7

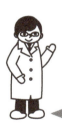

I have atopic dermatitis and my husband has a pollen allergy but no one in our families has asthma. I don't think she has inherited asthma. Do you think so?

Yes, it's possible.

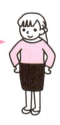

　母親が自分のアトピーや夫の花粉症を申告しつつも喘息の家族はいないので娘に喘息が遺伝しているとは考えていない旨を小児科医に伝え，Do you think so?　と確認していますが，医師は Yes. と親にアレルギーがあると子供に気管支喘息が出ることはありうることとまで言及しています。
　人は得てして自分の考えが絶対だと思い込みがちですが，さまざまな考え方があることを念頭に，この CS を活用しましょう。とくに相手が患者などの場合，医療従事者と異なった意見を言えない場合があることに配慮しましょう。

B Medical Reading

Medical Terminology

acute	急性の	hyperinflation	過膨張
airflow	気流	hypersensitivity	過敏
allergen	アレルゲン	IgE (Immunoglobulin E)	免疫グロブリンE
antagonist	拮抗薬	infantile	小児の
atmospheric pressure	気圧	leukotriene	ロイコトリエン
blood gas analysis	血液ガス分析（複数形は analyses）	mite	ダニ
		mold	カビ
bronchitis	気管支炎	obstruction	閉塞
carbon dioxide partial pressure	二酸化炭素分圧	peripheral	末梢の
		receptor	受容体
chronic	慢性の	respiratory	呼吸器の
dosage	1回投与量	smooth muscle	平滑筋
edema	浮腫	spirometer	スパイロメーター
emission rate	排出速度		
eosinophil	好酸球	steroid	ステロイド
expiration	呼気	stricture	狭窄
expiratory	呼気の	tract	管，道
house dust	ハウスダスト	$\beta 2$ stimulant	$\beta 2$ 刺激薬

Bronchial Asthma（気管支喘息）

Bronchial Asthma is a severe respiratory allergic response. The basic symptoms of bronchial asthma are chronic inflammation of the respiratory tract, airflow obstruction and respiratory hypersensitivity.

Inflammation in the respiratory tract caused by bronchial asthma induces edema in the bronchial smooth muscles or respiratory mucous membrane or develops into respiratory secretion, which causes stricture or obstruction. As a result, wheezing, shortness of breath, coughing or phlegm appears.

The symptoms tend to develop at night or early in the morning. Expiratory wheezing is characteristic of bronchial asthma. Extended expiration indicates worsening of the disease. It is a very dangerous state if the patient falls unconscious and the wheezing or breathing becomes weak.

Atopic asthma is characterized by inflammation indicating a type I allergy, most common in infants and young children. Infants often repeatedly wheeze from the age of two or three. Symptoms of infantile bronchial asthma may resemble those of bronchitis because respiratory tracts of young children are narrow and strictures are easily caused. Infantile asthma often disappears as the child matures though serious acute changes can become life threatening.

Allergens cause an allergic response. Allergens may include house dust, mites, pollen, mold, food, or medications. But other factors may also create an allergic response such as bacterial or viral infection, fatigue or stress, exercise, cigarettes, alcohol or changes of atmospheric pressure.

A respiratory function test using a spirometer shows a lowered emission rate of expiration. Partial pressure of carbon dioxide is lowered in mild cases and heightened in severe cases according to blood gas analyses. Chest X-rays show hyperinflation of lungs in acute cases. Blood tests show increasing eosinophil and nonspecific IgE in peripheral blood.

Inhalation steroid, $\beta 2$ stimulant, and leukotriene receptor antagonist are typical medication for bronchial asthma. The medicine and dosage are decided depending on the frequency and seriousness of the asthma attack.

Comprehension

1) 本文の内容について，次の問いに英語で答えなさい。

1. What are the basic symptoms of bronchial asthma?
2. What causes stricture or obstruction in asthma?
3. How might the symptoms of asthma become worse?
4. What are the danger signs of asthma?
5. What else can cause asthma besides allergens?
6. How does the emission rate of expiration change if one has asthma?
7. Why is it difficult to tell the cause of an infant's stricture?
8. How are medicine and dosage decided for bronchial asthma?

2) 本文の内容に合うように語群より適切な語句を選び，(　　) に入れなさい。

Inflammation by bronchial asthma leads to wheezing, shortness of (1), coughing or phlegm. Bronchial asthma is characterized by wheezing during (2). The condition of the disease can be seen by the length or emission (3) of expiration, the level of partial pressure of (4) dioxide, chest X-rays and conditions of eosinophil and nonspecific IgE in peripheral blood. Some of the important medications for asthma are Inhalation (5), β2 stimulants, or leukotriene receptor antagonists. Infant's stricture can be caused by either asthma or (6) and it is not easy to know which is the cause of the symptom. (7) of atopic asthma are house (8), mites, pollens, mold, food, medications etc. but other factors such as viral infection, fatigue or stress can bring the asthma attack. Children often get better as they get older, however, severe changes may be very dangerous.

carbon	bronchitis	dust	expiration	breath
allergens	rate	steroids		

ほっと一息！

「chronic ⇔ acute」のように医療分野でよく使われる対義語を覚えましょう。

peripheral 末梢の ⇔ central 中枢の
localized 局所の ⇔ generalized 全身の
congenital 先天性の ⇔ acquired 後天性の
benign 良性の ⇔ malignant 悪性の
expiration 呼気 ⇔ inspiration 吸気，または exhalation 呼気 ⇔ inhalation 吸気
primary 原発性の ⇔ secondary または sequential 続発性の
hypotension 低血圧 ⇔ hypertension 高血圧（hypo- ⇔ hyper-）

Helpful English Grammar

1．過去分詞の形容詞的用法

一般に動詞の過去分詞は「～された」という意味を表し，形容詞のように名詞・名詞句を修飾することがあります。（冠詞と）**過去分詞のみで修飾する場合**は名詞・名詞句の前に置き（例1，例2），さらに**長い語句とともに修飾**する場合は名詞・名詞句の後ろに置きます（例3）。

例1）**extended expiration**
　　引き伸ばされた呼気

例2）**a lowered emission rate of expiration**
　　低下した（低くされた）呼気排出速度

例3）**inflammation in the respiratory tract caused by bronchial asthma**
　　気管支喘息によって引き起こされた気道の炎症

2. 受動態

受動態は「**be 動詞＋過去分詞**」の形で「**～される**」という受け身の意味を表します。

Atopic asthma **is characterized** by inflammation….

アトピー性の喘息は炎症によって**特徴づけられる**。

Partial pressure of carbon dioxide **is lowered** in mild cases….

軽症では二酸化炭素分圧は**低下する（低くされる）**。

The medicine and dosage **are decided** depending on the frequency and seriousness of the asthma attack.

薬と投与量は，喘息発作の頻度や重症度により**決定される**。

ほっと一息！

この章では bronchus の複数形が bronchi であることを説明しましたが，このような不規則な複数形をもつラテン語系，古代ギリシャ語系の名詞が医療の分野では多く見られます。-us や -um の語尾のものでよく知られた語や医療で知っておきたい例をまとめました。

単数形の語尾が -us の形で，複数形の語尾が -i となる語

単数形	複数形	意味
bronchus	bronchi	気管支
fungus	fungi（funguses も使われる）	真菌類，菌類
stimulus	stimuli	刺激，激励
humerus	humeri	上腕骨
focus	foci（focuses も使われる）	焦点
octopus	octopi（octopuses も使われる）	タコ
radius	radii（radiuses も使われる）	半径
syllabus	syllabi（syllabuses も使われる）	概要，シラバス

単数形の語尾が -um の形で，複数形の語尾が -a となる語

単数形	複数形	意味
bacterium	bacteria	バクテリア，細菌
cranium	crania（craniums も使われる）	頭蓋，頭蓋骨
duodenum	duodena（duodenums も使われる）	十二指腸
ileum	ilea	回腸
jejunum	jejuna	空腸
rectum	recta（rectums も使われる）	直腸
ovum	ova	卵，卵子
perineum	perinea	会陰
serum	sera（serums も使われる）	血清，漿液

Chapter 13
Medication for a Young Child: Pharmacist

小児の薬物療法：薬剤師

　患者に薬について説明するのも薬剤師の重要な仕事です。小児やその母親と薬剤師の会話で，薬剤使用の目的，方法を母親に説明する表現を学ぶだけでなく，小児の理解を得るために積極的に小児とのコミュニケーションを図る例を学びましょう。そのほかにも，薬剤師には病院・診療所や調剤薬局等での処方箋に従った調剤，薬の開発のための研究などさまざまな活躍の場があることを読み取りましょう。

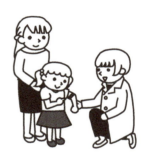

Purposes of this Chapter

臨床英語表現	貼付剤（貼り薬）使用に関連する表現
コミュニケーション・ストラテジー	相手の調子を尋ね，会話を始める
医療従事者の知識	薬剤師の資格，仕事についての正しい知識
重要構文	so that …, some … others … の構文

Medical Dialogue

Basic Medical Expressions

医療現場でよく使われる簡単な表現です。自然に言えるようになるまで声に出して何度も読み，完全に覚えましょう。

---

83 Be sure to dry the spot.
その場所をしっかり乾かしてください。

be sure to … は患者等に確実にしてもらいたい時に便利な表現です。

---

84 She may get a rash from the medicine.
彼女はその薬でかぶれるかもしれません。

「かぶれる」状態になることから動詞は get を使えます。

---

85 She has difficulty breathing.
彼女は呼吸困難になっています。

動詞 have で表せます。

---

86 Is there any other side effect I should be aware of?
その他に気をつけなければならない副作用はありますか？

医療従事者にとって side effect（副作用）は必修用語です。

Medical Terminology

limb	肢（腕，脚）	upper arm	上腕
side effect	副作用		

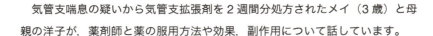

Medication for a Young Child（小児の薬物療法）

　気管支喘息の疑いから気管支拡張剤を2週間分処方されたメイ（3歳）と母親の洋子が，薬剤師と薬の服用方法や効果，副作用について話しています。

▅▷ 薬剤師は洋子と話をするために，メイにどのように話していますか。
▅▷ 洋子は薬の使い方について，何を理解したでしょうか。
▅▷ 最後（p.145-l.9）の薬剤師とメイとの会話はどのような効果があるでしょう。

In a meeting room in a hospital:

Hi. Look at this bandage. I had an injection.

 Oh, you had an injection? How are you?

I am a good girl. It hurt but I didn't cry.

She gave a blood sample for a test, not an injection.

 Oh, you gave blood for a test? You are a brave girl. Can you wait for a short while? I need to talk with your mother. Do you want to play with this toy monkey?

May starts playing with the toy:

 How are you feeling, Ms. Kato?

I am worried about her sickness.

 I understand how you are feeling. Let's help her recover together.

Yes. Do you think it is asthma?

I do not do diagnoses but the effects of this medicine may give us an idea. She can use this bronchodilator to expand her bronchi regularly for two weeks and see if her symptoms change.

 I see. I will help her take the medicine though she is not good at taking pills.

 Don't worry. The medicine is not a tablet or a capsule. It is a patch.

 That sounds easy!

 Yes, it is easy to use and you need to apply it only once a day.

 That's convenient. When should it be put on?

 She takes a bath in the evening, doesn't she?

 Yes. So I put it on after her bath.

 That's good timing. Be sure to dry the spot before you apply the patch.

 OK. Where should I put it on?

 You can apply it on her chest, back or upper arm.

 I think I should apply on her back so that she won't take it off.

That's a good place for a young child but don't apply it to the same position every day. She may get a rash from the medicine.

I see. Is there any other side effect I should be aware of?

 It rarely happens but if she has difficulty breathing or feels numbness in her limbs, remove the patch immediately and consult the doctor. Do you have any other questions?

No, I don't think so. Thank you.

The pharmacist turns to the girl to talk to:

 Good. Hi, May! Thank you for waiting. What a good girl you are!

I gave the monkey an injection.

 Oh, how is he feeling?

Not good. He coughs a lot.

 That's too bad. We can help him. How about giving him some medicine?

Okay. I will give him my medicine.

This is your medicine not his.

I don't like medicine.

This is different. You don't have to put it in your mouth. We just put this patch on.

Really?

Yes. Just put this on your back.

I will put it on the monkey's back.

 No, this is yours and I will give you medicine for the monkey.

Pharmacist takes out a seal:

 Here it is. This is his medicine. Would you put it on his back?

Can I? Good boy, monkey. I will give you your medicine. You get well! OK?

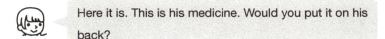 May, good job! You are like his mommy!

Mommy, will you put my medicine on my back?

Yes. I will after you have a bath.

Let's go home, Mommy.

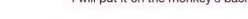 Good bye, May.

Bye-bye, monkey.

Thank you.

Additional Medical Expressions

87 She gave a blood sample for a test.
彼女は検査のために採血しました。
患者からいうと give blood となります。

88 You can apply it on her chest, back or upper arm.
彼女の胸，背中，上腕にそれを貼ることができます。

89 I would apply on her back so that she would not take it off.
彼女がそれをはがさないように背中に貼ります。
put on, apply に対して take off, remove

Let's Use Communication Strategies！

相手の調子を尋ね，会話を始める CS

簡単な挨拶も，習慣化しないとなかなか言えないものです。

p.142-l.7

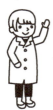
Hi. Look at this bandage. I had an injection.
Oh, you had an injection? How are you?
I am a good girl. It hurt but I didn't cry.

　薬剤師は，メイの自分の関心事を聞いてもらいたい気持ちを受け止めてから，定型の "How are you?" を使っています。それに対する答えは "I'm fine." などでなくてもいいでしょう。

p.142-l.14

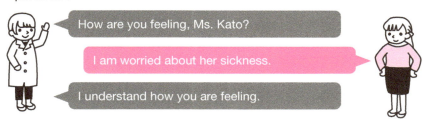

"How are you feeling?" や "How are you?" と聞かれた場合,いつでも "I'm fine." だとか,"I'm OK." と答えようと思わなくていいのです。その時の気分を状況に応じて答えられるといいですね。ただ,相手の状況を聞き出したら,それに気持ちを添えて言葉を返しましょう。

p.144-l.15

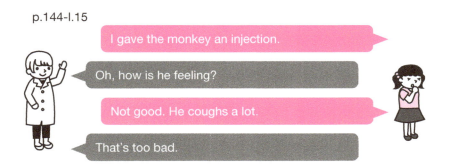

会話の相手にそれ以外の人の調子を尋ねる場合です。よく,ご家族の様子を "How is your mother?" などと聞きますね。

会話で良いスタートを切るために,自然に使えるように慣れましょう。

B Medical Reading

Medical Terminology

clinical testing	治験
dispense	調剤する
inpatient	入院患者

over-the-counter medicine	処方不要の市販薬
pharmaceutical	薬剤の
solution	液剤

Pharmacist（薬剤師）

Pharmacists work in various places: clinics, hospitals, pharmacies, drugstores, drug makers and so on.

In clinics and hospitals, pharmacists, as pharmaceutical specialists prepare medicines for outpatients and inpatients following prescriptions by doctors and they confirm the types and dosages prescribed by the doctor. They manage patients' pharmaceutical history and explain how to take the medicines so that patients use medicines effectively. Patients need to know the effects and the side effects to be expected in case they experience changes when taking the medicine. In many hospitals, pharmacists also prepare solutions for injections. To take proper care of patients, they need to cooperate with other medical specialists such as doctors, nurses, medical radiation technologists, registered dietitians, PTs, OTs and so on.

Pharmacists at dispensing pharmacies provide prescription drugs and necessary information about the medicine to outpatients of hospitals or clinics in the same way as the pharmacists in hospitals or clinics do. Since 1951, pharmacies have been allowed to be independent from doctors, although doctors in clinics and hospitals had been responsible historically both for treatment and administering drugs in Japan. Toward the end of the 20th century, many pharmacies started providing medicines with doctors' prescriptions. Pharmacists in drugstores without a prescription department are more independent selling over-the-counter medicines sometimes after consulting with customers on how to relieve their symptoms.

Many pharmacists work for drug makers in various capacities. Some study and experiment in a laboratory to discover or create new medicines. Others cooperate with doctors and researchers to certify the safety of new medicines, which is called clinical testing. There are also pharmacists who provide information about new medicines to doctors. Some pharmacists work with drug makers to promote their drugs.

Each job of a pharmacist is supported by specific knowledge and understanding of medicine. They need to study about medicine for six years at college and take a national examination to obtain a qualification as a pharmacist.

Comprehension

1）本文の内容について，次の問いに英語で答えなさい。
1. What do pharmacists do in clinics or hospitals?
2. Where else do pharmacists prepare medicines using prescriptions besides hospitals or clinics?
3. How does a pharmacist advise patients when they give medicines?
4. For proper care of the patient, who does a pharmacist cooperate with?
5. When was it first allowed for a dispensing pharmacist to give medicine following a doctor's prescription outside of the hospital?
6. Where does a pharmacist consult patients if they give medicines

without prescriptions?
7. Why do some pharmacists study or experiment in a laboratory?
8. How many years do they need to study to be a pharmacist?

2) 本文の内容に合うように語群より適切な語句を選び，(　　) に入れなさい。

　　Pharmacists are required in many workplaces. They give information to patients about effects and (1) of medicines and how to take medicines. Some pharmacists prepare medicines and solutions for (2) after they check if the medicine of doctor's (3) and the (4) are correct. Others sell (5) medicines consulting patients without doctor's prescriptions. In order to give medicines to patients properly, they need to know a patient's (6) history and they also need to tell patients what to expect if they take the medicines. Other pharmacists work to find or create a new medicine in a (7) or support doctors with (8) testing.

dosage	laboratory	side effects	over-the-counter
clinical	injections	prescriptions	pharmaceutical

Helpful English Grammar

1. ～ so that …

「…のように～」so that の後ろの節に can，may，could を使って「…できるように」とする文も多く見られます。

They … explain how to take the medicines **so that** patients use medicines effectively.

　彼らは患者が薬を効果的に使用する**ように**薬の服用法を説明する。

2. some … others …

「あるものは…他のものは…」と対照的に述べるときに使われます。

Some study and experiment in a laboratory. **Others** cooperate with doctors and researchers.

ある人たちは研究室で研究や実験をする。**他の人たちは**医師や研究者と協力する。

ほっと一息

カルテの記載方法

医療従事者はカルテの薬剤処方を正確に読み取る必要があります。わが国ではこれまでさまざまな方法による記載がなされてきたため、厚生労働省は平成22年1月に「内服薬処方せんの記載方法の在り方に関する検討会報告書」（http://www.mhlw.go.jp/shingi/2010/01/s0129-4.html）をまとめています。

従来の「1日分の薬物量を1日何回で分けて服用するか」という考え方に基づく記載方法は施設、医師等により多少違いはありますが、たとえば、「1錠が15mgのAという錠剤を1日に6錠、3回に分けて食後服用で7日分」処方する場合には「A（15）6錠分3毎食後7日分 n.d.E」あるいは「A錠15 mg 6T3×7日 n.d.E」などと記載がされます（Tはtabletの略で錠剤、カプセルであればcapsuleのC、顆粒や粉薬の包はpackのPで表します。n.d.Eはドイツ語の略語で食後、v.d.Eは食前、z.d.Eは食間、v.d.Sは就寝前を表します）。

同じ処方内容でも上記報告書の記載方法に従うと、「分量」の記載は「最小基本単位である1回量を記載することを基本」とされることから「A錠15 mg 1回2錠1日3回 朝昼夕食後7日分」となります。

Chapter 14
Acupuncture and Acupuncturist

鍼灸と鍼灸師

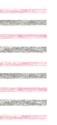

　腰痛のため鍼灸院を訪れている様子を会話例で学びましょう。

　鍼灸は2千年以上の歴史があり，治療は長年の実践，経験に基づいて行われています。昨今では鍼灸師は東洋医学の知識のみならず，西洋医学の知識をも習得し，慢性疾患なども鍼ともぐさで治療をしています。さらに，最新の機器を使用しサイエンスとして鍼灸治療効果を分析するようになっています。

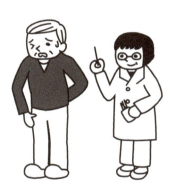

Purposes of this Chapter

臨床英語表現	鍼灸の治療に関連する表現
コミュニケーション・ストラテジー	相手の発言内容について説明を求める
医療従事者の知識	鍼灸についての正しい知識
重要構文	関係代名詞の所有格　the 名詞 of which，by ＋動名詞，助動詞 must，by ＋再帰代名詞

Medical Dialogue

Basic Medical Expressions

医療現場でよく使われる簡単な表現です。自然に言えるようになるまで声に出して何度も読み，完全に覚えましょう。

---

90 My lower back pain is killing me.
腰痛がひどい。
腰痛の医学専門用語は lumbago

---

91 My condition is worse than yesterday.
昨日より調子が悪いです。

---

92 I will take your pulse.
脈をとります。
pulse beat は脈動；感情（意向）を示します。

Medical Terminology

a strained back	ぎっくり腰	Meridian	経絡
acupuncture treatment	鍼治療	needle	鍼（鍼治療では「鍼」の漢字を使用する）
holistic	全体的な，全人的な（holistic medicine：全人医療）	Oriental Medicine	東洋医学
lower back pain	腰痛	ouch!	あうっ，痛い（突然の鋭い痛みに対する叫び）
		summarizing	要するに

Acupuncture（鍼灸）

一郎（65歳）が昨日，夏野菜を植えるために畑を耕している最中，急に腰が痛くなり，動けなくなりました。今朝もまだ腰が痛くて動くことができませ

ん。一郎の状態は昨日より悪化しているようです。京子（25歳）が心配しているため、健（32歳）が一郎の様子を見に来ました。

▶ 鍼治療はどんな症状に最も効果がありますか？
▶ 鍼灸師はどのように一郎の状態を確認しますか？
▶ 鍼灸治療における経絡とはどのようなものですか？
▶ 「全人的」とは何を意味していますか？

Ken: Good morning, Ichiro. How is your lower back pain?

Ichiro: Good morning, Ken. My lower back pain is killing me. My condition is worse than yesterday.

Kyoko: That's too bad. Do you know how to relieve Ichiro's pain, Ken?

Ken: I have read articles in some journals that acupuncture treatment works for pain the best. Recently some diseases are being treated with acupuncture in the US and Europe as well as in China.

Kyoko: I have read the article, too. Moreover, WHO recognizes acupuncture treatments for several kinds of diseases.

Ichiro: Ouch! I have never been experienced this kind of pain before.

Ken: You should go to the acupuncture clinic as soon as possible today. I know a good acupuncture clinic, so I will make an appointment.

Summarizing, acupuncture treatment is the best for my lower back pain. I want an acupuncturist to relieve my pain as soon as possible.

At the acupuncture clinic:

Good morning, is this your first time visiting us?

Yes, I have got a strained back and terrible lower back pain which prevents me from moving and walking now.

Please fill in this medical sheet and be seated here until you are called.

At the consulting room:

Good morning, Mr. Kato. According to your medical sheet, you have lower back pain now, don't you?

Yes, I got a strained back yesterday. My lower back pain is much worse than yesterday.

I will check your whole body. Please put out your tongue.

What do you mean? I have a trouble with my lower back, not my tongue or mouth.

I know. We understand a patient's body condition by checking the color and shape of his or her tongue.

Really? That's surprising.

Now, let me take your pulse.

Pulse? Could you explain? Why do you take pulse for lower back pain?

 Acupuncture treatment is the major part of Oriental Medicine, in which the idea of Meridian is the most important.

Meridian? The line connects the North Pole and the South Pole? What do you mean?

 The Meridian of acupuncture is a channel of the life power flow (qui). A bad point of the body is connected with some other points on the Meridian running through the body. Therefore we must cure not only the patient's bad point but the patient's whole body. This idea is called a "holistic view".

I am interested in acupuncture, but I am afraid of being treated with a needle.

 Don't worry. You will neither feel pain nor bleed because the needle for treatment is thinner than a hair.

I am relieved to hear what you say.

Ichiro's lower back pain got much better thanks to acupuncture treatment and he could walk to his house on that day. He has got acupuncture treatment once a week in order to keep a healthy body condition since then.

Additional Medical Expressions

(93) Acupuncture treatment works for pain the best.
鍼灸治療は痛みに一番よく効きます。
work：効き目がある

(94) I have got a strained back.
ぎっくり腰になった。
strained back：ぎっくり腰　strain：無理をしてだめにする，（筋などを）違える

Let's Use Communication Strategies !

相手の発言内容について説明を求める CS

相手の言った内容を納得できないときには，どう返したらよいでしょう。

p.155-l.17

Please put out your tongue.

What do you mean? I have a trouble with my lower back, not my tongue or mouth.

　鍼灸師が舌を出すように言ったのに対し，一郎は腰が痛いのになぜ舌を診るのか疑問に思って「どういうことですか？」と尋ねています。

p.156-l.2

Now, let me take your pulse.

Pulse? Could you explain? Why do you take pulse for lower back pain?

鍼灸師が脈を取ろうとするのに，一郎は腰痛で脈を取る理由を「説明してもらえませんか？」と尋ねています。

p.156-l.8

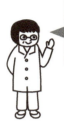

Acupuncture treatment is the major part of Oriental Medicine, in which the idea of Meridian is the most important.

Meridian? The line connects the North Pole and the South Pole? What do you mean?

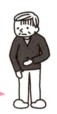

鍼灸師が Meridian（経絡）の考えが一番重要だと説明するのに対し，一郎は Meridian を地球の経線だと思っているので，意味がわからず「どういう意味ですか？」と尋ねています。

このように言葉としては聞き取れていても，内容が理解できないときには "What do you mean?" "Could you explain?" などの CS で説明を求めることができます。わからないことは放置しないで，尋ねて理解するようにしましょう。

Medical Reading

Medical Terminology

acupuncture point	つぼ	Five Elements Theory	五行説
advocate	提唱する	indisputable	明白な
conflict	対立する，衝突する	living body reaction	生体反応
construct	組み立てる，〜を構成する	material world	物質世界
		moxa	もぐさ

Moxibustion	灸治療	the kinetic system	運動系
natural phenomena	自然現象 (phenomenonの複数形)	the nervous system	神経系
		theoretical system	理論体系
stiff shoulder	肩こり	Traditional Chinese Medicine	伝統中医学
the digestive system	消化器系	Yin and Yang Theory	陰陽理論

Acupuncture and Moxibustion（鍼灸）

　Acupuncture and Moxibustion is one of major treatments of Traditional Chinese Medicine (TCM), the history of which began more than two thousand years ago. The theory was established by experiences and practicing that many people had practiced for a long time. The ancient great people described the relation between natural phenomena and body's internal phenomena in the old books of Oriental Medicine. They also advocated human beings as a part of nature. The main theoretical system consists of the "Yin and Yang Theory" and the "Five Elements Theory". The former theory is that "Yin" shows dark, cold and quiet in the natural world while "Yang" shows light, warmth and noise. Both of them depend on and conflict with each other. The "Five Elements Theory" shows five important substances in the material world: wood, fire, earth, metal and water. These five substances are indisputable to daily lives. Both Nature and human beings are constructed by movable change of these five substances.

　Acupuncturists treat a patient's bad body condition by inserting thin needles into a patient's body and stimulating acupuncture points that exist on 360 points through the body. They sometimes use moxa, which is put on acupuncture points and burned for the purpose of warming a patient's body and causing his or her living body reaction. Acupuncturists diagnose a patient's body condition with four diagnose methods, that is to say, "望 (bou), 聞 (bun), 問 (mon), 切 (setu)": "bou" means watching, "bun" means listening or smelling, "mon" means asking, and "setu" means touching. Acupuncturists also diagnose with their five senses and examine a patient's whole body.

The Japanese have an image that acupuncture treatment especially effects on stiff shoulders and lower back pain. However, WHO announced acupuncture treatments are effective for 43 diseases which include the diseases of the nervous system, the digestive system and the kinetic system.

In an aged society, acupuncture treatment is paid much attention because it is effective for preventing illness and keeping a healthy condition.

Acupuncturists must study both Western and Eastern Medicine for three or four years at training school or university. In Japan there are 11 universities and 111 training schools for developing acupuncturists. After finishing schooling, they take a national examination to get a national license. Acupuncturists can open their own clinic and diagnose and treat patients by themselves. Nowadays acupuncture treatment is undergone in 160 countries in the world and more and more clinical researches are being done to demonstrate how acupuncture works on several diseases. It is necessary for acupuncturists to acquire much medical knowledge for working as a member of a team of medical staff.

Comprehension

1) 本文の内容について，次の問いに英語で答えなさい。
1. When did the history of Traditional Chinese Medicine begin?
2. What does the main theoretical system of Oriental Medicine consist of?
3. What do "Yin" and "Yang" show?

4. How does an acupuncturist diagnose a patient?
5. How many acupuncture points are there on the body?

2) 本文の内容に合うように語群より適切な語句を選び，(　　) に入れなさい。

Acupuncture and Moxibustion is one of major treatments of (1) that has a history going back more than two thousand years. The ideas of the treatment have been enriched by practicing of many people through many periods. The main theoretical system consists of the (2) and the "Five Elements Theory", which are theories based on the diagnose methods. Acupuncturists view patients as (3) using their five senses and treat patients with needles and moxa. The way of taking the patient's whole body is called a (4). It is getting more important to examine his or her whole body because diseases are more likely to be (5) and interconnected with other diseases.

| chronic | Yin and Yang Theory | Traditional Chinese Medicine |
| a whole body | holistic view | Western Medicine |

Helpful English Grammar

1. the 名詞 ＋ of which：関係詞の所有格を表す

先行詞が人以外の場合，関係代名詞の whose に加え of which が使われます。
Acupuncture and Moxibustion is one of major treatments of Traditional Chinese Medicine, **the history of which** began more than two thousand years ago.
鍼灸は伝統中医学の主要な治療の一つで，**その歴史**は二千年以上前に始まりました。
That is a book **whose title** is popular among the young.

That is a book, **the title of which** is popular among the young.
　あれは若者の間で人気のタイトルの本です。

2. by ＋ 動名詞：〜することによって
Acupuncturists treat patients' bad body condition **by inserting** thin needles into patients' body.
　鍼灸師は患者の体に鍼を刺す**ことによって**体の不調を治療する。
The patient got better by being treated in the hospital.
　患者は病院で治療して**もらうことによって**よくなった。

3. 助動詞　must：〜しなければならない
Acupuncturists **must** study both Western and Eastern Medicine at university or training school for three or four years.
　鍼灸師は3年または4年間，大学もしくは専門学校で東洋医学と西洋医学の両方を勉強**しなければならない**。

・**助動詞の後には動詞の原形**がきます。重要な助動詞には以下があります。
　can：〜することが可能である，〜かもしれない
　may：〜してよい，〜かもしれない
　must：〜しなければならない，〜に違いない
　should：〜するべきだ，〜のはずだ

4. by ＋再帰代名詞：独立して，一人で
Acupuncturists can open their own clinic and diagnose and cure patients **by themselves**.
　鍼灸師は自分の治療院を開き，**自分で**患者を診断，治療することができます。
Did you do the work by yourself?
　あなたは**自分で**その仕事をしたのですか？

・再帰代名詞：I → myself, we → ourselves, you → yourself (yourselves), he → himself, she → herself, it → itself, they → themselves

・**再帰代名詞の重要表現**

take care of yourself：お身体をお大事に

help yourself to ～：～をご自由にお取りください

talk to oneself：独り言をいう

enjoy oneself：楽しくすごす

ほっと一息！

Q 鍼灸治療が肩こり，腰痛に効果があると聞いています。医療雑誌で「WHOが鍼灸治療効果がある疾患を認めている」とありましたが，どんな疾患が認められているのですか？

A 以下に「WHO（世界保健機構）で鍼灸療法の有効性を認めた病気」の一覧を示します。最近ではがんの疼痛，食欲不振にも鍼治療がされています。ぜひ参考にしてください。

【神経系疾患】◎**神経痛**・神経麻痺・痙攣・脳卒中後遺症・自律神経失調症・頭痛・めまい・不眠・神経症・ノイローゼ・ヒステリー

【運動器系疾患】関節炎・◎**リウマチ**・◎**頚肩腕症候群**・◎**頚椎捻挫後遺症**・◎**五十肩**・腱鞘炎・◎**腰痛**・外傷の後遺症（骨折，打撲，むちうち，捻挫）

【循環器系疾患】心臓神経症・動脈硬化症・高血圧低血圧症・動悸・息切れ

【呼吸器系疾患】気管支炎・喘息・風邪および予防

【消化器系疾患】胃腸病（胃炎，消化不良，胃下垂，胃酸過多，下痢，便秘）・胆嚢炎・肝機能障害・肝炎・胃十二指腸潰瘍・痔疾

【代謝内分秘系疾患】バセドウ病・糖尿病・痛風・脚気・貧血

【生殖，泌尿器系疾患】膀胱炎・尿道炎・性機能障害・尿閉・腎炎・前立腺肥大・陰萎

【婦人科系疾患】更年期障害・乳腺炎・白帯下・生理痛・月経不順・冷え性・血の道・不妊

【耳鼻咽喉科系疾患】中耳炎・耳鳴・難聴・メニエール病・鼻出血・鼻炎・ちくのう・咽喉頭炎・へんとう炎

【眼科系疾患】眼精疲労・仮性近視・結膜炎・疲れ目・かすみ目・ものもらい

【小児科系疾患】小児神経症（夜泣き，かんむし，夜驚，消化不良，偏食，食欲不振，不眠）・小児喘息・アレルギー性湿疹・耳下腺炎・夜尿症・虚弱体質

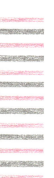

Chapter 15
Hemodialysis: Interdisciplinary Team Approach to Medicine

血液透析：チーム医療

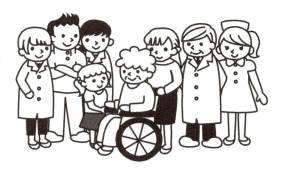

　血液透析開始までには，シャント作成を含め透析についてさまざまな視点から重要な説明がなされます。透析を開始することとなった患者と看護師との会話から，多くの医療従事者がチームで関わる状況を学びましょう。

　このように医療の専門職がチームで協力する体制は，日本では「チーム医療」といわれますが，これに当たる固定的な英語表現はないようなので，interdisciplinary team approach to medicine としました。

Purposes of this Chapter

臨床英語表現	血液透析開始に備えたシャント作成に関連する表現
コミュニケーション・ストラテジー	相手の発言内容について説明を求める
医療従事者の知識	チーム医療の背景と役割についての正しい知識
重要構文	過去完了形と現在完了進行形の構文

Medical Dialogue

Basic Medical Expressions

医療現場でよく使われる簡単な表現です。自然に言えるようになるまで声に出して何度も読み，完全に覚えましょう。

95
Did you understand the doctor's explanation?
医師の説明はわかりましたか？

動詞 explain の名詞が explanation。

96
Do you have any other questions?
他にご質問はありますか？

相手が質問しやすいように，こうした表現を使ってみてください。

97
Follow the advice of our experts.
私たち専門家の助言に従ってください。

「従う」には follow を使っています。

Medical Terminology

certified social worker	社会福祉士	shunt	シャント
clinical engineer	臨床工学技士	subsidy	補助金
dialysis	（血液）透析	urologist	泌尿器科医
interdisciplinary	学際的な	urology	泌尿器科

Hemodialysis（血液透析）

糖尿病による腎障害のため，血液透析を開始するためのシャントを作成することになった三浦日紗子（69歳）と泌尿器科看護師が，泌尿器科医師の診察後に話し合っています。

▶ 日紗子は医師の説明をどのように理解しているでしょうか。

■▷ 日紗子はこのあと，どのような医療従事者と会うことになりますか。
■▷ 多くの医療従事者と会う目的はそれぞれ何でしょう。

After a consultation with a urologist:

 Nurse: Hi. Did you understand the doctor's explanation?

 Hisako: Yes, I think so. My kidneys can't purify the blood well which brought on my various symptoms and gave us the poor results for my blood test. I need to clean up my blood through a machine.

 That's right. You need hemodialysis through a dialysis machine.

 Yes, hemodialysis. And I will have an operation to make a thick blood vessel for hemodialysis?

 You are right. A shunt for hemodialysis will be created in the operation.

 Yes, I will need a shunt and have hemodialysis. Is it two times or three times per week?

 You have to come to the dialysis department three times per week.

 It means 12 or 13 times per month. How much will it cost to have a hemodialysis?

 The medical fees for the treatment are very expensive but you may be able to receive subsidies for that.

That's why I will talk with a social worker this afternoon?

 Yes. A certified social worker will visit you this afternoon.

OK. How long does it take each time for the dialysis?

 It usually takes four or five hours. A nurse in the dialysis department will explain in detail. Do you have any other questions?

Well, I want to know about the mechanism for hemodialysis.

 OK. I will call a clinical engineer for an explanation.

Clinical engineer?

 Yes. They are specialists in medical devices.

There is a specialist in medical devices? I haven't heard of any expert's name.

 Don't worry. You can see him before the nurse in the operation room comes to explain about the operation. Do you have any other questions?

Can I eat meat after I start dialysis? I eat so little now.

 That's a difficult question. You will have an opportunity to talk with a registered dietitian after the operation.

OK. A certified social worker, a clinical engineer, nurses in an operation room and dialysis department and a registered dietitian … Anyone else?

 And a pharmacist will explain about your medication.

I am so popular!

 Yes, many people want to see you! We are treating you as a medical team.

Everybody in the team sounds like an expert in their field.

 That's right! We are medical specialists in an interdisciplinary team.

I feel at ease with your support as a team.

 Yes, we will be behind you all the way. So please be careful in your daily life and follow the advice of our experts.

OK.

Additional Medical Expressions

A shunt for hemodialysis will be created in the operation.
手術で透析のためのシャントが作られます。
will be ＋過去分詞で受動態の未来形です。

You may be able to receive subsidies for that.

99 そのための補助金を受けることができるかもしれません。

補助金が必ず受けられると決まっていないので may を用いています。

We are medical specialists in an interdisciplinary team.

100 私たちは専門家の医療チームです。

inter は「相互の」交流があることを意味し，disciplinary は「学問分野の」という意味なので各専門分野の専門家が協働する医療チームであると覚えておいてください。

Let's Use Communication Strategies !

相手の発言内容を簡単にまとめて確認する CS

相手の言った内容を自分の言葉で言い換える CS は難しいかもしれませんが，自分の理解を相手に伝えて共通の認識を深め，会話を発展させます。

p.166-l.9

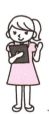

… My kidneys can't purify the blood well which brought on my various symptoms and gave us the poor results for my blood test. I need to clean up my blood through a machine.

That's right. You need hemodialysis through a dialysis machine.

患者の理解を聞いて，看護師が簡潔に言い直しています。患者に難解な専門用語を使うことは避けるべきですが，hemodialysis はそれほど難しい単語ではないため，今後の治療に便利だという看護師の判断かもしれません。

p.166-l.13

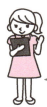

…And I will have an operation to make a thick blood vessel for hemodialysis?

You are right. A shunt for hemodialysis will be created in the operation.

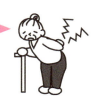

患者の理解内容は正しいのですが，今後便利なので，シャントという語を覚えてもらいたいのかもしれません。

p.168-l.10

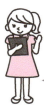

Everybody in the team sounds like an expert in their field.

That's right! We are medical specialists in an interdisciplinary team.

医療チームの皆が各領域の専門家のようだという患者に，各学問分野にまたがるチームであると看護師が伝えることで安心感を与えることができているようですね。

このように，相手の言っている内容を言い変えてその妥当性をさらに補完したり，副産物的に相手に便利な表現を紹介したり，時には微調整していくことも可能なこのCSが使えると，会話はさらに深まることでしょう。

B Medical Reading

Medical Terminology

complement	補足する
pyramid	ピラミッド

speech and swallowing therapy	言語聴覚療法
standardization	標準化

Interdisciplinary Team Approach to Medicine（チーム医療）

Doctors had been located on the top of medical workers' pyramid for a long time in Japan. They had been responsible for various problems concerning patients' treatment: nursing care, nutrients, medication, physical therapy, occupational therapy, speech and swallowing therapy, dental therapy, medical devices, X-rays, laboratory tests, social welfare, mental support etc. Rather than a pyramid, recent illustration for medical staff is a circle including doctors around a patient in the center. Each field in medical service has been developing remarkably and medical workers need to study new information and skills in specific courses in schools. Doctors also have been learning more complicated medical sciences each year and need to depend on experts of other fields.

Medical staff required in the clinical field had been obedient hard workers following the doctors' directions. Nowadays, they need to perform their accurate judgments based on their knowledge and technology complementing other staff's approach. Therefore, obtaining better knowledge and technology with confidence, they share information and experience with the team. Through clear communication with other staff, they understand others' ways of thinking and asserting their informed viewpoints in a collaborative exchange.

In this condition, each medical worker has to be above a certain level of competence to be a specialist in their field. To certify their levels, most of medical fields prepare tests for the candidates after they have studied in specific colleges or schools for a certain period. Even after passing the tests, they still need to acquire the latest information to discharge their responsibility as specialists. Therefore, they become reliable experts for patients and other medical staff including doctors due to their improving knowledge or skills. This condition is the basis of the interdisciplinary team approach to medicine.

Medical specialists in the interdisciplinary team share their knowledge, information and responsibilities by cooperating and complementing each other. To improve the quality of interdisciplinary team approach to medicine, standardization of the medical service and team management based on communication and cooperation are important. Therefore, they need not only to exchange information but also discuss and coordinate their performances so that they can best treat their patients and improve their chances of recovery.

Comprehension

1）本文の内容について，次の問いに英語で答えなさい。

1. Until recently for what kind of issues had doctors been responsible?
2. Why do medical staff need to study more in each field?
3. How can medical specialists keep their levels high?
4. Why can we trust in the knowledge and skills of a medical specialist?
5. What do medical specialists in a team share by cooperating and complementing each other?
6. How else besides exchanging information can the medical specialists in a team improve their patients' chances of recovery?

2）本文の内容に合うように語群より適切な語句を選び，（   ）に入れなさい。

Doctors had to deal with everything concerning a (1) in the past in Japan. They had to manage (2), nutritionists, (3), physical therapists, occupational therapists, speech therapists, dental hygienists, clinical engineers, social workers, clinical psychologists and so on. These medical workers, however, need (4) and newer (5) and technologies and they have studied to be certified as (6) in each field. Doctors still are a very important part of the medical team; however, they can rely on other (7) and vice versa. Patients are treated cooperatively and complementally with this (8) team. The team aims to perform better medical service by improving team standards and management.

staff	nurses	knowledge	interdisciplinary
better	patient	specialists	pharmacists

ほっと一息！

職業とその業務や学問を表す語を確認しましょう。

職業を表す語	業務や学問を表す語の例
医師　doctor/physician	medicine, medical science
看護師　nurse	nursing, nursing care
臨床検査技師　medical technologist	clinical laboratory examination
管理栄養士　registered dietitian	dietetics, nutrition science
理学療法士　physical therapist	physical therapy
診療放射線技師　medical radiation technologist	medical radiation technology, radiography, radiation medicine
薬剤師　pharmacist	pharmacy, pharmacology
作業療法士　occupational therapist	occupational therapy
鍼灸師　acupuncturist	acupuncture treatment

Helpful English Grammar

1. 過去完了形

「**had ＋過去分詞**」の形で過去のある時点までの継続，経験，完了，結果を表します。

They **had been** responsible for various problems concerning patients' treatment.

　彼らは患者の治療に関するさまざまな問題について責任を**問われてきていた**。

Medical staff required in the clinical field **had been** obedient hard workers.

　臨床分野に求められる医療スタッフは，従順で勤勉な働き手**であった**。

2. 現在完了進行形

「**have（has）＋ been ＋〜ing**」の形で，過去から現在まで継続してきており，現在も進行していることを表します。

Each field in medical service **has been developing** remarkably.

　医療サービスの各領域は著しく**発展し，現在も発展している**。

Doctors also **have been learning** more complicated medical sciences.

　医師はまた，より複雑な医療科学を**学んできており，なお継続的に学んでいる**。

ほっと一息！

　この章で「血液透析」hemodialysis という単語を覚えましたが，その構造は hemo ＋ dialy ＋ sis だと気づきましたか？

hemo-　　「血液」の意味（hem-, haem- も同意）
dialy-　　「分離した」の意味

-sis 　　「過程，活動」（病的な状態の意味で使われることも多い）

今回は接頭辞 hemo- と接尾辞 -sis に注目して医療現場で覚えておきたい語を紹介します。このようなところから語彙を豊かにしたいですね。

接頭辞 hemo-/hem-/haem- の語彙例
hematemesis（吐血）　　　hemoptysis（喀血）
hematocrit（赤血球容積率）　hemorrhage（大出血）
hemoglobin（ヘモグロビン）　hemorrhoid（痔）
hemophilia（血友病）

接尾辞 -sis「過程，活動」の意の語彙例
analysis（分析）　　　　homeostasis（ホメオスタシス）
genesis（発生）　　　　metastasis（がん細胞などの転移）

接尾辞 -sis「病気」の意の語彙例
amyloidosis（アミロイド症）　nephrosis（ネフローゼ）
acidosis（アシドーシス）　　neurosis（神経症，ノイローゼ）
alkalosis（アルカローシス）　osteoporosis（骨粗しょう症）
cyanosis（チアノーゼ）　　paralysis（麻痺）
ketosis（ケトーシス）　　　sclerosis（硬化症）
lipidosis（脂肪代謝異常）　thrombosis（血栓症）
narcosis（昏睡）　　　　　tuberculosis（結核）

Comprehension 解答

Chapter 2

1) 1. Influenza viruses do.
   2. They are a high fever, chills, shivering, a cough, a headache, body aches, fatigue and reddened eyes and face.
   3. It takes 15 minutes.
   4. Tamiflu capsule or Inavir Dry Powder Inhaler is.
   5. The news of the appearance of a new influenza virus which is tolerant of Tamiflu capsule and human beings' infection of bird influenza does.

2) 1. flu
   2. coughing
   3. nasal secretion
   4. headache
   5. fatigue
   6. being diagnosed

Chapter 3

1) 1. It shows that nurses have four responsibilities to accomplish their duties: promotion of health, prevention of disease, restoring of health, and relief of pain.
   2. He built a monastery and advocated the importance of medicine.
   3. He conducted research into beriberi and founded the first training school in Japan.
   4. It was changed in 2003.
   5. More medical knowledge and special technology focused in advanced medicine are.

2) 1. My cousin who lives in Sendai is a nurse.
   2. A nurse is always busy taking care of patients every day.
   3. My aunt is in the hospital. She is taken care of by a nurse well at the hospital.

Chapter 4

1) 1. The accumulation of triglyceride by taking much fats and sugar in liver cells is.
   2. Hepatitis A virus is transmitted orally. Hepatitis B and C viruses are transmitted by blood.
   3. It is likely to spread from winter to the beginning of spring, especially in March and April.
   4. They are fever, symptoms of cold, general fatigue, loss of appetite and nausea.
   5. It is fulminant hepatitis.

2) 1. inflammation
   2. blood
   3. GPT
   4. sugar liquid
   5. fulminant hepatitis
   6. hepatitis A virus vaccination

Chapter 5

1) 1. They primarily work in a laboratory.
   2. Red blood cells or white blood cells are examined.
   3. They cultivate samples to detect the existence of some microbes.
   4. The tissues from our organs are examined.
   5. An electrocardiogram, electroencephalogram, pulmonary function test, electromyogram, funduscopy, ultrasound and magnetic resonance imaging are examples of physiological function tests performed by MTs.
   6. They have to study at least three years.

2) 1. urine
   2. digestive
   3. proteins
   4. bacteria
   5. antigens
   6. genes
   7. transfusions
   8. transplants

Chapter 6

1) 1. They are type A diabetes mellitus, type 2 diabetes mellitus, gestational diabetes mellitus and other type of diabetes mellitus.
   2. They are obesity, stress and not enough exercise.
   3. They diagnose by the result of the examinations such as fasting plasma glucose level, 75 g oral glucose tolerance level and HbA1c.
   4. Type 1 diabetes occurs among infants and young people by absolute insulin deficiency. While type 2 diabetes occurs among the middle aged people. It is related to obesity and life-style factors.
   5. They are diet treatment, exercise treatment and medical treatment.

2) 1. increased thirst
   2. weight loss
   3. a blood vessel
   4. diabetic neuropathy
   5. diabetic retinopathy
   6. diet treatment
   7. exercise treatment

Chapter 7

1) 1. They are taking care of sick and wounded people and keeping food safety standards and quality for meeting nutritional requirements.
   2. He or she can get a license of RD by two ways. One way is to have the national qualification examination of RD while educating people about nutrition with a dietitian license. The other is to have the examination of RD after graduating from university or training school admitted as an institution for training a registered dietitian.
   3. He or she works in the medical facilities, elderly welfare facilities, community and educational facilities.
   4. He or she makes a menu for diabetes, kidney disease, cardiovascular disease, obesity, osteoporosis etc.
   5. He or she offers knowledge about food for babies or elderly people.

2) 1. 厚生労働省
   2. 管理栄養士養成指定
   3. 傷病者
   4. 専門知識
   5. 在宅療養

Chapter 8

1) 1. Pathological fracture might often occur in the elderly.
   2. Repeatedly imposed stresses on certain areas cause stress fracture.
   3. It is classified as incomplete fractures.
   4. It is called an open (compound) fracture.
   5. The open (compound) fracture is most at risk for infection.
   6. The typical procedure is to reset the bones to their natural positions and immobilize them in a cast for about four weeks.
   7. It is to prevent contracture or CRPS caused by the immobilization of the joint in the cast.

2) 1. pathologic
   2. simple fracture
   3. compound fracture
   4. reset
   5. cast
   6. rehabilitation

Chapter 9

1) 1. They are to relieve a patient's pain experienced when they move.
   2. Most PTs work in hospitals, clinics, nursing facilities, assisted living facilities, adult day-care centers and clients' homes.
   3. They work with elderly people and disable children to keep or promote their ADL as well as with healthy people or athletes to provide methodology for safe and effective training.
   4. They perform manipulating passive movements of joints, muscle massage, traction therapy, electrotherapy, ultrasound therapy, warming or icing etc.

5. They must study three or four years before taking the national exam.
6. He/she should have a variety of knowledge. For example, they need to learn the anatomy and physiology of the human body and diseases, internal medicine, orthopedic surgery and understanding their clients' mental state.

2) 1. disabled
   2. mobility
   3. improve
   4. relieve
   5. joint
   6. massage
   7. minds
   8. national

Chapter 10

1) 1. They are primary and metastatic lung cancers.
   2. It occurs within the cells of lung tissues.
   3. Primary lung cancer is most common.
   4. A surgical operation is important to treat it.
   5. A squamous cell carcinoma is the most related to smoking.
   6. Lung cancer gives the highest death rate of all the cancers.
   7. Smoking, air pollutants and occupational related dust are risk factors for primary lung cancers.

2) 1. 原発性
   2. 遺伝子
   3. 喫煙
   4. 危険因子
   5. 扁平上皮
   6. 腺
   7. 血流

Chapter 11

1) 1. They are to provide and interpret digital image scans for a doctor's diagnosis and treatment or to give radiation treatments to patients with malignant tumors.
   2. All organs and regions of the human body are targeted by X-rays.
   3. He/she would take X-rays of the chest to detect lung or heart diseases or an accidentally swallowed foreign object.
   4. We can find images of gas in the intestines, ulcers or cancers.
   5. Computed tomography does.
   6. They are called contrast enhanced CT scans and simple CT scans.
   7. Angiography is a contrast enhanced CT.
   8. The advantage of MRI is that it does not have radiation exposure.
   9. Ultrasonography does not need a large device as CT or MRI does.

2) 1. 診断
   2. 肺炎
   3. 腸閉塞
   4. 誤飲
   5. 骨シンチグラフィ
   6. 単純
   7. 造影
   8. 血管造影
   9. 被曝
   10. 超音波

Chapter 12

1) 1. The basic symptoms of bronchial asthma are chronic inflammation of the respiratory tract, airflow obstruction and respiratory hypersensitivity.
   2. Inflammation induced edema in the bronchial smooth muscles develops into respiratory secretions causing stricture or obstruction.
   3. The symptoms worsen into wheezing, shortness of breath, coughing or production of phlegm.
   4. Unconsciousness and weakened wheezing or breathing are danger signs of asthma.
   5. Bacteria or viral infection, fatigue or stress, exercise, cigarettes, alcohol or changes of atmospheric pressure can also cause asthma.
   6. It becomes lower.
   7. Young children have narrow respiratory tracts and strictures are easily caused, so symptoms of infantile bronchial

asthma may resemble those of bronchitis.
8. They are decided depending on the frequency and seriousness of the asthma attack.

2) 1. breath
   2. expiration
   3. rate
   4. carbon
   5. steroids
   6. bronchitis
   7. allergens
   8. dust

Chapter 13

1) 1. They prepare medicines for outpatients and inpatients following prescriptions by doctors and they confirm the types and dosages prescribed by the doctor.
   2. They prepare them at dispensing pharmacies.
   3. They explain how to take medicines, the effects and the side effects of the medicines.
   4. He/she cooperates with other medical specialists such as doctors, nurses, medical radiation technologists, registered dietitians, PTs, OTs and so on.
   5. It was first allowed in 1951.
   6. A pharmacist consults patients in the drugstores.
   7. They work in a laboratory to discover or create new medicines.
   8. They need to study for six years to be a pharmacist.

2) 1. side effects
   2. injections
   3. prescriptions
   4. dosage
   5. over-the-counter
   6. pharmaceutical
   7. laboratory
   8. clinical

Chapter 14

1) 1. It began more than two thousand years ago.
   2. It consists of the "Yin and Yang Theory" and the "Five Elements Theory".
   3. "Yin" shows dark, cold, and quiet in the natural world. "Yang" shows light, warmth and noise in the natural world.
   4. He or she diagnoses a patient with four diagnose methods: "bou", "bun", "mon" and "setu".
   5. There are 360 acu points.

2) 1. Traditional Chinese Medicine
   2. Yin and Yang Theory
   3. a whole body
   4. holistic view
   5. chronic

Chapter 15

1) 1. They had been responsible for various problems concerning patients' treatment: nursing care, nutrients, medication, physical therapy, occupational therapy, speech and swallowing therapy, dental therapy, medical devices, X-rays, laboratory tests, social welfare, mental support etc.
   2. They need to study more because each field in medical service has been developing remarkably.
   3. They keep their levels high by studying new information even after they pass the qualifying tests.
   4. We can trust due to their improving knowledge or skills.
   5. They share their knowledge, information and responsibilities.
   6. Discussing and coordinating their performances can improve their patients' chances of recovery.

2) 1. patient
   2. nurses
   3. pharmacists
   4. better
   5. knowledge
   6. specialists
   7. staff
   8. interdisciplinary

英文索引

A

abdominal pain 8
acetaminophen 18
acupuncture point 158
acupuncture treatment ... 153
acupuncturist.................... 28
acute................................ 134
acute appendicitis 34
acute hepatic disease 34
acute viral hepatitis 39
adult day-care center 98
affect................................. 87
alcoholic liver disease 39
allergen 134
allergic 8
allergy 129
anatomy............................ 98
anemia............................... 51
anesthesia 82
antagonist....................... 134
antibody............................ 18
anticancer drug 105
antigen.............................. 51
antipyretic 13
antiviral drug.................... 13
appetite 34
armpit 24
assisted living facility........ 98
asthma................................ 8
atmospheric pressure..... 134
atopic.............................. 129

B

bacteria............................. 51
bend 93
beriberi 28
bile 39
blood gas analysis........... 134
blood tests........................ 34
blood transfusion................ 8
blood vessel 124
bloody stool....................... 8
bone tumor 87
bronchi 112
bronchial......................... 129
bronchitis........................ 134

C

carcinoma...................... 112
cast................................... 82
Celsius 2
cerebral........................... 124
certified social worker 165
cervix 18
chemotherapy 105
chest pain 8
chill 8
chilly 13
chronic............................ 134
clinical engineer.............. 165
clinical testing................. 148
compatibility 51
complication..................... 57
constipation....................... 8
contaminated water......... 39
contracture 87
contraindicate.................. 18
crack................................. 87
cultivate 51

D

dermatitis........................ 129
diabetes....................... 8, 62
diabetic diet..................... 70
diagnose 13
diagnosis 34
dialysis 165
diarrhea.............................. 8
diet therapy 70
digestive 51
disabled............................ 98
dispense 148
dizziness............................. 8
dizzy 117
dosage............................ 134
dose 13
drowsy............................ 117
drug administration 28
duodenum 124

E

edema............................. 134
elbow 82
electrotherapy 98
Employees' Health
    Insurance 2
eosinophil 134
epidemic........................... 19

F

epithelial 112
esophagus...................... 124
expiration....................... 134
exposure......................... 124

F

Fahrenheit.......................... 2
family history 105
fasting glucose level......... 57
fatigue................................ 8
fatty liver disease............. 39
feces................................. 39
feel weak 8
feeling of fullness............. 70
fever convulsion 19
fracture 82
frequent urination 57
fulminant hepatitis 39

G

gauze................................ 45
gene................................. 51
general anesthesia 105
general fatigue................. 13
general hospital 2
general physical weariness 8
geriatric food 76
germ 51
gestational diabetes mellitus
    62

H

health insurance card 2
hemodialysis.................... 62
hemorrhage 124
hepatitis virus 39
high blood pressure........... 8
holistic 153
hormone 51
house dust..................... 134
hyperinsulinemia.............. 62
hypersensitivity.............. 134
hypertension...................... 8

I

ideal body weight 70
IgE 134
ileus 124
immobilize 87
immunity.......................... 19
Inavir dry powder inhaler.. 19

incision 105
incubation period.............. 39
indisputable 158
infantile 134
inflammation 39
influenza 13
inhalation 13
inherited 129
injection 45
inpatient........................... 148
insulin resistance 62
interdisciplinary 165
internal medicine 8
intestinal tract................... 39
intestine 124
invasive.............................. 51

J・K・L
joint pain 8
kidney 8
Langerhans island 62
limb 141
liver 8
living tissue........................ 51
locomotive syndrome 98
lower back pain 153
lymph node...................... 105

M
magnetism....................... 124
malignant 51
manifestation 39
manipulate........................ 82
medical examination report
 57
medical radiation
 technologist................... 51
medical sheet 8
medical technologist 45
menopause.......................... 8
Meridian.......................... 153
metastasis 105
metastatic....................... 112
microbe 51
midwife 28
mite.................................. 134
mold 134
moxa................................ 158
Moxibustion.................... 159
muddled 117
muscle pain 13

mutation 112

N
nasal discharge 13
National Health Insurance .. 2
nausea 8
needle 153
nephropathy 57
numbness............................ 8
nursing facility 98

O
obesity 76
obstruction 134
oral glucose tolerance test
 57
Oriental Medicine 153
orthopedics 82
osteoporosis 76
outpatient 8
ovary 124
over-the-counter medicine
 148

P・Q
painkiller 82
painless 117
palpitation........................... 8
pancreas........................... 62
pediatric........................... 129
period 8
peripheral 134
pharmaceutical............... 148
pharmacist........................ 28
pharynx............................. 19
phlegm................................ 8
physical therapist 28
physiological..................... 51
physiology 99
pneumonia.......................... 8
pollutant.......................... 112
poor appetite 8
positive rate 39
prescribe............................. 8
prognosis.......................... 39
protein 51
public health nurse 28
pulmonary...................... 124
pulmonary function test.... 51
QOL 99

R
radiation.......................... 124
radiation treatment 105
radiologist......................... 28
radiology......................... 117
rash..................................... 8
receptor 134
recur 105
red blood cell.................... 51
reference............................. 2
registered dietitian............ 28
rehabilitation 83
relieve 99
reset.................................. 83

S
sample 45
shivering 19
shortness of breath 8
side effect 141
sleep disorder................... 24
sluggish 2
smooth muscle............... 134
sore throat 8
specimen 51
speech and swallowing
 therapy 171
sterile 45
steroid............................. 134
stiff 93
stiff shoulder................... 159
sting 45
strained back.................. 153
stretch 93
stricture 134
stroke.................................. 8
survival rate 106
suspected diabetes........... 57
swab 13
symptom 8

T
tablet 13
Tamiflu capsule................. 19
the digestive system....... 159
the kinetic system 159
the Ministry of Health, Labor
 and Welfare 76
the nervous system 159
theoretical system 159
therapeutic 99

181

thermometer 24	運動療法 70	血液検査 34
tolerance 87	X線 83	結核 8
trachea 112	炎症 39	血管 124
tract 134	嘔吐 8	月経期間 8
transplant 51	悪寒戦慄 19	血便 8
tuberculosis 8	汚染水 39	解熱剤 13
	汚染物質 112	解熱鎮痛剤 18
U		下痢 8
ulcer 124	**か行**	健康診断報告書 57
uncomfortable 13	介護老人保健施設 98	健康保険 2
upper arm 141	解剖学 98	言語聴覚療法 171
urinary 124	潰瘍 124	倦怠 8
urination 8	外来患者 8	検体 45, 51
urology 165	化学療法 105	高インスリン血症 62
uterus 124	華氏 2	抗ウイルス薬 13
	ガーゼ 45	抗がん剤 105
V	画像 105	高血圧 8
vaccination 39	家族歴 105	抗原 51
vein 45	肩こり 159	好酸球 134
virus 13	脚気 28	拘縮 87
vomiting 8	合併症 57	厚生労働省 76
	カビ 134	抗体 18
W・X	過敏 134	更年期 8
welfare facility 99	管 134	呼気 134
white blood cell 51	がん 112	呼吸機能検査 51
wrist 83	肝炎ウイルス 39	国民健康保険 2
X-ray 83	寒気 8	骨腫瘍 87
	関節痛 8	骨折 82
	肝臓 8	骨粗しょう症 76
	管理栄養士 28	固定する 87
	気圧 134	
和文索引	気管 112	**さ行**
	気管支 112	細菌 51
	気管支炎 134	再発する 105
あ行	ぎっくり腰 153	肢 141
悪性の 51	ギプス 82	磁気 124
アトピー性の 129	急性ウイルス性肝炎 39	子宮 124
アルコール性肝炎 39	急性肝炎 34	市販薬 148
アレルギー 129	急性虫垂炎 34	しびれ 8
アレルゲン 134	灸治療 159	脂肪肝 39
息切れ 8	吸入 13	社会福祉士 165
移植 51	狭窄 134	十二指腸 124
痛む 45	胸痛 8	出血 124
イナビル吸入剤 19	禁忌 18	受容体 134
インスリン抵抗性 62	筋肉痛 13	障がいのある 98
インスリン分泌 57	空腹時血糖 57	消化器系 159
咽頭 19	くび 18	錠剤 13
咽頭痛 8	軽減する 99	症状 8
インフルエンザ 13	経口ブドウ糖負荷試験 57	小児科（学）の 129
ウイルス 13	経絡 153	上皮の 112
運動系 159	劇症肝炎 39	静脈 45

上腕	141
食事療法	70
食道	124
食欲	34
食欲不振	8
助産師	28
処置する	82
処方する	8
神経系	159
腎臓	8
診断	13, 34
診療放射線技師	51
睡眠障害	24
ステロイド	134
整形外科	82
生存率	106
生体	51
整復する	83
生理学的な	51
切開	105
赤血球	51
摂氏	2
全人医療	153
全身倦怠感	8, 13
全身麻酔	105
喘息	8
潜伏期間	39
卒中	8

た行

体温計	24
耐性	87
ダニ	134
タミフルカプセル剤	19
だるい	8
痰	8
胆汁	39
タンパク質	51
治験	148
注射	45
腸	124
腸管	39
調剤する	148
腸閉塞	124
鎮痛剤	82
デイケアセンター	98
適合性	51
転移	105
転移性の	112
電気療法	98
伝染病	19

動悸	8
透析	62, 165
糖尿病	8, 62
糖尿病予備軍	57
東洋医学	153
突然変異	112

な行

内科	8
入院患者	148
ネフロパシー	57
脳の	124
伸ばす	93

は行

肺炎	8
排尿	8
肺の	124
ハウスダスト	134
吐き気	8
白血球	51
発症	39
発疹	8
鼻水	13
鍼治療	153
肘	82
微生物	51
泌尿器の	124
被曝	124
皮膚炎	129
肥満	76
病原菌	51
貧血	51
頻尿	57
不快な	13
副作用	141
福祉施設	99
腹痛	8
浮腫	134
不調の	2
平滑筋	134
閉塞	134
便	39
便秘	8
放射線	124
放射線技師	28
放射線療法	105
保健師	28
ホルモン	51

ま行

麻酔	82
末梢の	134
慢性の	134
満腹感	70
無菌の	45
めまい	8, 117
免疫	19
免疫グロブリンE	134
問診表	8

や行

薬剤師	28
輸血	8
陽性率	39
腰痛	153
予後	39
予防接種	39
与薬	28

ら行

卵巣	124
理学療法士	28
理想体重	70
リハビリテーション	83
臨床検査技師	45
臨床工学技士	165
リンパ節	105
老人食	76
老人福祉施設	98
ロコモティブ症候群	98

編著者紹介

髙木久代（1～4, 6, 7, 14章）
鈴鹿医療科学大学 保健衛生学部 教授

小澤淑子（5, 8～13, 15章）
鈴鹿医療科学大学 看護学部 教授

著者紹介

矢田　公（8, 10章）
鈴鹿医療科学大学 医用工学部長

西村　甲（12章）
鈴鹿医療科学大学 保健衛生学部 教授

小林由直（2, 4, 6章）
三重大学 保健管理センター 准教授

NDC490　191p　21cm

チーム医療のためのメディカル英語　基本表現100

2015年2月20日　第1刷発行
2020年2月3日　第5刷発行

編著者	髙木久代・小澤淑子
著　者	矢田　公・西村　甲・小林由直
発行者	渡瀬昌彦
発行所	株式会社 講談社

〒112-8001　東京都文京区音羽2-12-21
　　　販売　(03) 5395-4415
　　　業務　(03) 5395-3615

編　集	株式会社 講談社サイエンティフィク
	代表　矢吹俊吉

〒162-0825　東京都新宿区神楽坂2-14　ノービィビル
　　　編集　(03) 3235-3701

本文データ制作	株式会社 エヌ・オフィス
カバー表紙印刷	豊国印刷 株式会社
本文印刷・製本	株式会社 講談社

落丁本・乱丁本は，購入書店名を明記のうえ，講談社業務宛にお送りください．送料小社負担にてお取替えいたします．なお，この本の内容についてのお問い合わせは，講談社サイエンティフィク宛にお願いいたします．定価はカバーに表示してあります．

© H. Takagi, Y. Kozawa, I. Yada, K. Nishimura and Y. Kobayashi, 2015

本書のコピー，スキャン，デジタル化等の無断複製は著作権法上での例外を除き禁じられています．本書を代行業者等の第三者に依頼してスキャンやデジタル化することはたとえ個人や家庭内の利用でも著作権法違反です．

JCOPY　〈(社)出版者著作権管理機構 委託出版物〉

複写される場合は，その都度事前に(社)出版者著作権管理機構（電話 03-5244-5088，FAX 03-5244-5089，e-mail: info@jcopy.or.jp）の許諾を得てください．

Printed in Japan
ISBN 978-4-06-155624-9